Pain Management

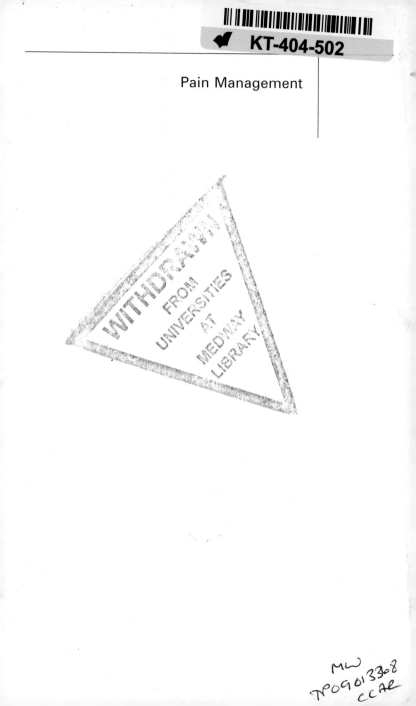

Pain Management

Eileen Mann
BSc (Hons), RGN, SCM, PGCHE
Nurse Consultant, Poole Hospital NHS Trust and
Lecturer, Institute of Health and Community Studies,
Bournemouth University

AND

Eloise Carr
BSc (Hons), RGN, PGCEA, RNT, MSc, PhD
Reader, Institute of Health and Community Studies,
Bournemouth University

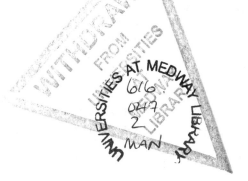

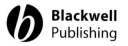

Blackwell
Publishing

© 2006 Eileen Mann and Eloise Carr

Blackwell Publishing Editorial offices:
Blackwell Publishing Ltd, 9600 Garsington Road, Oxford OX4 2DQ, UK
  Tel: +44 (0)1865 776868
Blackwell Publishing Inc., 350 Main Street, Malden, MA 02148-5020, USA
  Tel: +1 781 388 8250
Blackwell Publishing Asia Pty Ltd, 550 Swanston Street, Carlton, Victoria
3053, Australia
  Tel: +61 (0)3 8359 1011

First published 2006 by Blackwell Publishing Ltd

ISBN-10: 1-4051-3071-7
ISBN-13: 978-1-4051-3071-4

Library of Congress Cataloging-in-Publication Data
Mann, Eileen M.
Pain management / Eileen Mann, Eloise Carr.
   p. ; cm.
Includes bibliographical references and index.
ISBN-13: 978-1-4051-3071-4 (pbk. : alk. paper)
ISBN-10: 1-4051-3071-7 (pbk. : alk. paper)
1. Pain.   2. Pain–treatment.   I. Carr, Eloise C. J.   II. Title.
[DNLM: 1. Pain–classification.   2. Pain–therapy.   3. Palliative Care.
WL 704 M2816p 2006]
RB127.M36 2006
616'.0472–dc22
2005037641

A catalogue record for this title is available from the British Library

Set in 9/11 pt Palatino
by SNP Best-set Typesetter Ltd., Hong Kong
Printed and bound in Singapore
by Markono Print Media Pte Ltd

For further information on Blackwell Publishing, visit our website:
www.blackwellnursing.com

Contents

Foreword

The publication of this volume could not be more timely. Earlier this year the International Association for the Study of Pain (IASP) brought out the second edition of their outline curriculum on pain for nursing. It provides a framework for pre-registration nurses, identifying the essentials that should be learned about pain; a nurse should be able to identify the patient who has pain, assess the pain and its impact, initiate action to alleviate or manage the pain and evaluate the effectiveness of any action.

This sounds simple enough but we know from numerous studies (some of which are mentioned in *Pain Management*) that many people have unrelieved pain at home and – possibly worse – in hospital. This pain may be due to an underlying disease or trauma, we may find no pathology to explain it, or it may be acute or persistent, but one thing is certain – it will be having an effect on the person experiencing it and those around them. Our understanding of pain has changed in the last 40 years and we now view it from a biopsychosocial perspective. This bringing together of the various components of pain means we should no longer think of one treatment approach; assessment and management will be multi-faceted.

Nurses are in a unique position to facilitate good pain management. We see the patient in different environments, interacting with various people, and spend more time with them than most other healthcare professionals. Good pain management requires an interdisciplinary approach and nurses have ready access to other healthcare professionals. But we cannot provide this care if the basic knowledge and skills in understanding, assessing and managing pain are not in place.

Eileen Mann and Eloise Carr have provided us with these tools in *Pain Management*. Considering pain in different stages of life, the authors acknowledge the clinical challenges we face and provide practical suggestions. Learn them, practice them and apply them to become a nurse who not only understands the effect pain may have, but is also knowledgeable and confident in helping people manage it.

Ruth Day
Consultant Nurse
Peterborough & Stamford Hospitals NHS Trust

Preface

Welcome to the first edition of *Pain Management* which forms part of the *Essential Clinical Skills for Nurses* series.

This book provides information and guidance on pain management through a lifetime, recognising that as we develop and age our experiences of pain may change. Nurses often have the privilege of being able to be with the patient over long periods of time. This provides an ideal opportunity to assess pain, select appropriate interventions and deliver therapeutic clinical skills.

We are more susceptible to pain at different times in our life and this inevitably impacts on our psychological well-being and social life. To reflect the diversity of pain and to assist in the development of clinical skills, we have arranged this book in chapters that cover pain commonly experienced from childhood through to old age. In some instances, where pain experiences are not exclusive to a specific age group, we have tried to select those that are most common for that particular age group. Different types of pain are described within each chapter with examples of evidence-based therapeutic management, where these exist, as well as resources that can help in clinical judgement. In addition web links are given to patient self-help groups and other educational resources.

There are two notable exclusions from the book. The first is the management of pain in palliative care and the second is the management of pain during pregnancy and childbirth. Traditionally these have been viewed as specialist subjects in their own right. They also represent growing fields of research and practice. As a result we feel they are beyond the scope of this book.

As an introduction the first chapter discusses some of the mechanisms of acute and chronic pain, describing the current theories that relate to these mechanisms. The second chapter expands on these theories and helps to describe the different types of pain that may be experienced and discusses the basic principles of pain management.

Subsequent chapters cover pain through the lifespan, giving case histories to help illustrate real life situations and how these may be managed to optimise pain control.

We hope you will enjoy this format and find the text, illustrations and tables informative and easy to use. Ultimately we hope the book gives you the confidence to combine the knowledge and skills to deliver effective nursing care to those who experience pain.

Eileen Mann
Eloise Carr

Acknowledgements

We would like to thank Clive Andrewes and Di Halliwell at the Institute of Health and Community Studies, Bournemouth University, for providing the intellectual environment and support to complete this endeavour.

We would also like to acknowledge the staff at Poole Hospital NHS Trust for their innovation and desire to try new ways of working. We are particularly grateful to Dr. Barry Newman, Mandy Layzell and Polly Cameron of the Acute Pain Team for their contributions and to Martin Smits (Director of Nursing) and Yvonne Jeffrey (Deputy Director of Nursing) for their encouragement.

A special thank you must also be given to Susan Merner from the library at Poole Hospital NHS Trust whose skill navigating databases and finding elusive articles never let us down. Thank you to Vivian Maiden and Sian Jenkins for their helpful suggestions with the chapters associated with pain in children.

As always, a big thank you must also be given to both our husbands Peter and Tim, especially Peter, whose mastery of computer illustration has proved invaluable in enhancing the quality of the text. He so generously gave his time.

Glossary of Terms

Afferent: nerves that transmit messages from the periphery to the central nervous system (CNS)

Allodynia: pain felt from what would normally be a simple touch sensation such as stroking the skin

Autonomic: the part of the nervous system that is not under conscious control, such as regulation of the heart and digestion

Breakthrough pain: pain over and above background pain that is not being relieved by current analgesia, usually associated with moving a damaged limb, coughing following abdominal surgery or pressure on injured tissues, etc.

Causalgia: pain that is described as burning and is associated with nerve damage

Central pain: pain associated with a disturbance or malfunction within the CNS, i.e. the spinal cord and the brain

Cutaneous pain: pain associated with a painful stimulus or a painful lesion on the skin

Efferent: the nerves that transmit messages from the CNS to the periphery

Endorphines: morphine-like analgesics that are produced naturally in the CNS

Hyperalgesia: increased sensitivity to a painful stimulus

Idiopathic pain: this describes pain that despite intensive investigation appears to have no definable origin or related pathology

Incident pain: this is really another term for breakthrough pain but is also used to describe pain that is associated with interventions that can sometimes cause considerable pain, such as some treatments, diagnostic procedures and dressing changes. Because the pain caused may only last for a short period analgesia is frequently overlooked or simply not considered

Limbic system: part of the brain that processes emotional responses and behaviour and is closely associated with the experience and interpretation of pain

Molecule: in this instance molecules refer to particles that are released and transmit information from one cell to the other, thereby passing messages up to and down from the brain and spinal cord. These may be hormones or neurotransmitters, e.g. serotonin, potassium ions, inflammatory mediators such as bradykinin and endorphins

Neurogenic pain: pain arising from nerves themselves rather than nerve activity as a response to painful stimulation

Neuropathy: a disturbance of nerve function, which may be sensory loss, altered sensation or pain

Nociceptor: a nerve that responds to potentially painful stimuli

Radiculopathy: pathology in the area of a nerve root

Referred pain: this is simply pain felt in an area that is different from the site of pathology. It is associated with how the nervous system developed in fetal life. It means nerve pathways may be shared by nerves coming from organs and peripheral tissues that are actually quite far away from each other. The brain then struggles to locate the accurate source of the pain. Typical referred pain would be a heart attack being felt as pain in the left shoulder and arm

Substantia gelatinosa: the jelly-like area that is found within the dorsal horn of the spinal cord and represents an area of intense synaptic activity associated with the processing of pain

Understanding the Principles of Pain Management

1

'Pain is perfect misery; the worst of evils, and excessive overturns of patience.' John Milton, *Paradise Lost*

INTRODUCTION

The experience of pain permeates the world of every living soul. It can cause remorseless suffering and does not discriminate across age or class. This chapter explores definitions and describes the neurophysiology necessary to accurately assess and manage pain, before briefly reviewing pain theories which have evolved to explain this unpleasant experience. It is essential that these concepts are understood, as they are fundamental to the assessment and management of the person in pain. We cannot endorse this enough. This chapter forms the foundation upon which the book is built, with a particular focus on the sensory, psychological and social components of pain. You may need to refer back to this chapter, the following chapter and the glossary at regular intervals.

LEARNING OBJECTIVES

❏ To outline the mechanisms of acute and chronic pain
❏ To describe current theories that relate to the mechanisms of these pains
❏ To discuss the impact of pain on individual experience
❏ To give an overview of assessment and evaluation

WHAT IS PAIN?

Can you describe what pain is? Words such as 'hurt' and 'discomfort' come to mind and it is also unpleasant. In 1968 Margo McCaffery defined pain as 'whatever the experiencing person says it is and existing whenever he says it does' (McCaffery 1968). This is helpful as it emphasises believing the person and what he or she says about his or her pain. In 1979, the International Association for the Study of Pain (IASP) introduced the most widely used definition of pain, which was published in the journal *Pain* in 1986 (IASP 1986). IASP defined it as '**an unpleasant sensory and emotional experience associated with actual or potential tissue damage, or described in terms of such damage**'. This is helpful but it does not explain how pain can be felt even when there appears to be no tissue damage, such as the pain associated with a stomach cramp or appearing to come from a phantom limb. There are situations where victims have experienced immense tissue damage but do not appear to be in pain. Pain is a private and subjective experience, which can only be felt by the person experiencing it.

UNDERSTANDING ACUTE PAIN

Neurophysiology

This section will explore how the sensation of pain, from **pain receptors**, is conveyed along specific pain fibres called **nociceptors**. The neural transmission of nociceptive impulses can be modulated through a variety of **transmitting** molecules.

It is important to understand the basic neurophysiology involved in the sensation of pain. Any stimulation that has the potential to cause damage to skin or tissue may cause us to experience pain. This stimulation might be from a sharp object that cuts the skin, fascia and muscle during surgery or a blunt implement that may bruise tissue or break bone. Heat and fire may burn or scald, as can the chemicals released from a bee or nettle sting. The result is an unpleasant sensation, which draws our attention to where we perceive the sensation is coming from. This is acute '**first pain**' and it informs us that something has happened and we need to do something about it. People born with a rare genetic disorder that renders them unable to perceive pain rarely live to adulthood as they are robbed of these warning signs of impending tissue damage and are unable to seek medical help or take evasive action.

Pain receptors

Pain receptors are present throughout the body, especially the skin, surfaces of the joints, periosteum (the specialised lining around the bone), arterial walls and certain structures in the skull. Some organs have less pain receptors (gut, muscle, etc.). It is interesting to note that the brain itself does not have any pain receptors at all, and is therefore insensitive to any potentially painful stimuli inflicted on it.

There are three types of pain receptor:

- Mechanical
- Thermal
- Chemical

A mechanical stimulus (touch) would be, for example, high pressure or stretch, and a thermal pain stimulus would be extreme heat or cold. Chemical pain receptors can be stimulated by chemicals in the outside world (e.g. acids), but also by certain products that are present in the body and locally released upon trauma or inflammation or other painful stimuli.

Pain fibres

The mechanisms responsible for the sensation or 'sensory' component of pain are now described. From peripheral sites around the body, such as the skin and intestine, sensations are transmitted to the spinal cord and from there to the brain by sensory nerve fibres. Sensory nerve fibres have various functions and come in a variety of sizes. They also vary in how quickly their messages reach the brain. There are three types of nerve fibres that are of particular interest to us:

- A-delta fibres
- C fibres
- A-beta fibres

These **afferent** sensory fibres synapse at the spinal cord and impulses are transmitted up the spinal cord to the brain.

The A-delta fibres respond to mechanical or thermal stimulation, e.g. a pin prick or scald. They are fast because they are covered in an insulation layer called myelin and warn of impending tissue damage. Your quick reaction when you touch a hot hob on the cooker is a response to stimulation of these fibres. C fibres are sometimes referred to as polymodal as they respond to thermal, mechanical and chemical stimulation; they are slower fibres that transmit the dull, thudding pain of injury, inflammation or disease. The A-beta fibres transmit touch and play a very important role in the sensation of pain, which is explained later in this chapter.

All the fibres travel to the **dorsal horn** of the spinal cord, which is divided up into layers of cells called **laminae**. These laminae have been numbered according to location. Most finish in lamina I and II. The nerves then give off long fibres, which cross to the other side of the cord and travel up to the **thalamus** and **somatosensory** areas of the brain cortex. The A-delta fibres end in the 'thinking' part of the cortex which is why we can accurately locate where the pain is. Interestingly these fibres are also responsible for pinprick sensation. A patient who has been given a strong dose of morphine for pain will still jump if his or her skin is pricked. This is a protective mechanism and very difficult to abolish unless the patient is deeply anaesthetised or a nerve block is used. Adequate analgesia to help control background pain can aid in an accurate assessment and prove helpful in diagnosis.

Case study

John had been admitted in the morning to the surgical ward with acute abdominal pain, localised in his right iliac fossa. A preliminary examination by the junior doctor suggested that he probably had appendicitis. John was placed on the operating list for later in the day. Despite being in severe pain, which John described as 'knife like and burning', no opioid analgesia was prescribed as the junior doctor was concerned that it might mask John's underlying condition and was waiting for the senior registrar to examine him. John lay curled up facing the wall as still as possible.

This situation is totally unnecessary and not unusual. Strong analgesics (e.g. opioids such as morphine) will not mask the 'first pain' and therefore should have been given for his severe pain. When John was examined the 'first pain' was still intact as a protective mechanism to ensure the tissue was not exposed to further damage. Patients should not be left in such pain.

The C fibres are slower than the A-delta fibres in their conduction and are associated with '**second pain**'. That is the dull, burning, aching, throbbing pain which is generally diffuse over a wide area usually after the initial sharp pain. It may occur minutes or hours later.

A-beta fibres, whilst they do not transmit pain sensation, are part of the larger picture. They occur in the skin and are the largest of the three fibres. While they synapse in the dorsal horn they do not cross over in the spinal cord and are the fastest conducting. These fibres are activated by touch and cutaneous stimulation which can be used therapeutically (see Table 1.2).

Case study

Jane was running to catch the bus yesterday when she tripped on a paving stone and twisted her ankle. She felt a sharp tearing sensation and sudden acute pain. Hobbling home she put an ice pack on the ankle and took a couple of painkillers. The pain was very sharp and localised. The next morning when she woke up she could hardly move her ankle and the whole area was swollen and sore.

Can you identify from this case study which fibres might be responsible for the different experiences?

Nociceptive inputs from viscera and muscle are poorly localised. This means the sensation of pain is quite diffuse and cannot be pinpointed to a localised area. This is because the synapse from these fibres does not terminate in the substantia gelatinosa (lamina II) but in lamina I and IV.

Pain chemicals

Chemicals have a vital role to play in the transmission of pain. Injury or trauma naturally produces an 'inflammatory soup' and, rather like an exotic minestrone, it has many different chemical ingredients. The principal ones are **substance P**, **bradykinin** and the **leukotrienes**. They are very important as they play a major role in a 'chemical cascade', which ultimately causes the inflamed tissue and surrounding area to become increasingly sensitised to pain by the production of **prostaglandins**, particularly prostaglandin E.

Table 1.1 Neurotransmitters involved in the transmission of pain within the central and peripheral nervous systems.

Neurotransmitter	Location	Action
Amino acid		
Glutamate	Central nervous system: brain and spinal cord	• Most widely found excitatory neurotransmitter in the CNS
Peptides		
Endorphins	Central nervous system: brain and limbic system	• Endogenous opiate 'morphine-like': 'runner's high', 'tears of joy after childbirth' • Inhibits substance P and thus inhibits pain
Substance P	Central nervous system: basal ganglia and mid brain Peripheral nervous system: sensory neurons	• Neurotransmitter of pain-responsive neurons
Somatostatin	Central nervous system: hypothalamus and pancreas	• Neurotransmitter of the enteric nervous system
Cholecystokinin	Central nervous system: cerebral cortex and small intestine	• Neurotransmitter of the enteric nervous system

Substance P is a peptide neurotransmitter that is involved in pain signals, and is found (among other places) in the type-C fibres of peripheral nerves that carry pain signals to the central nervous system. It is also released in the dorsal horn of the spinal cord as a response to painful stimulation. Other excitatory amino acids include glutamate, somatostatin and cholecystokinin (Table 1.1).

Damaged cells from any sort of trauma release a vast soup of chemicals, which initiate the firing of nerve cells involved in the transmission of pain and actually make the nerve more sensitive to further stimulation. This might account for pain appearing to get worse several hours after injury as the inflammatory process becomes well established.

It has long been recognised that trauma to any tissues is often accompanied by an area of hypersensitivity surrounding the trauma. This is sometimes called **secondary hyperalgesia** to distinguish it from the increased sensitivity to pain within the trauma area known as primary hyperalgesia. Hyperalgesia is recognised by an increase in pain produced by stimuli at the threshold for pain or by a decrease in the pain threshold in that area.

Following an injury or trauma, dorsal horn cells are bombarded by stimuli originating from pain receptors. Over a period of time, the receptive field of these cells increases. While it is likely that many chemical processes are involved in central sensitisation, N-methyl D-aspartate (NMDA) receptors are thought to be key in the process. This process of increasing central sensitisation of dorsal horn cells has been called **wind up**.

Theories to explain the experience of pain

The previous sections have hopefully built a picture of the structures and transmitters involved in the experience of pain. They are just the start of the story and by no means explain the entire experience of pain seen in clinical practice. From this background we can understand how acute pain is perceived and why the different nerve fibres give rise to different sensations – fast pain and secondary or slow pain. There is more. Here are some of the anomalies, which cannot easily be explained:

- On the battlefields of the Second World War it was observed that significant numbers of men who had lost limbs did not require morphine for their pain (Beecher 1959).
- Some people experience excruciating pain when there appears to be no apparent injury.
- Chronic pain sometimes persists long after the original injury has healed.
- Some patients become extremely sensitive to the lightest of touch, which can produce very distressing pain.

One of the main theories of pain was that offered by Descartes in the seventeenth century and called the **specificity theory**. A philosopher influenced by science, he proposed that the body worked like a machine and injury provoked specific pain receptors, which sent messages to a pain centre in the brain. It was a very unforgiving model and made no allowances for all the psychological factors known to influence our perception of pain. It is mentioned because the fallout of this theory continues to influence today.

In 1965 Ronald Melzack and Patrick Wall brought together their physiological and psychological knowledge to propose a theory, which would prove to be one of the most powerful and enduring theories of pain. It was known as the **gate control theory**. Some key components and implications for clinical practice are listed below in Table 1.2.

The gate control theory changed the way in which pain was thought about and indeed managed. The two important aspects, which explained so much, related to the descending modulation at the dorsal horn level and the dynamic role of the brain in pain

Table 1.2 The gate control theory and clinical implications.

Gate control theory	Clinical implications
• The transmission of nerve impulses from afferent fibres to the spinal cord transmission (T) cells is modulated by a spinal cord gating mechanism.	Due to this, 'modulation' volleys of pain impulses traveling up the spinal cord might be amplified or decreased, thus altering the experience of pain.
• The gating mechanism is influenced by the activity in A-beta fibres and C fibres.	The small C fibres conveying the sharp pain facilitate transmission or 'open the gate'. The A-beta fibres inhibit transmission or close the gate. The use of cutaneous stimulation for the management of pain illustrates this, e.g. rubbing one's shin after walking into a coffee table.
• The spinal gating mechanism is influenced by nerve impulses descending from the brain.	The role of fear, anxiety and maybe anger can modulate the experience of pain. The use of relaxation strategies and psychological interventions are recognised as important interventions.
• Large diameter rapidly conducting fibres activate selective cognitive processes that then influence, by way of descending fibres, the modulating properties of the spinal gating mechanism.	Sensory input can modulate pain. Patients report pain being worse at night due to lack of sensory input. The use of distraction techniques, music and a variety of sensory rich therapies can influence the experience of pain.

processing. **Descending modulation** has important implications for the management of pain (Fig. 1.1).

The brain is capable of releasing neurotransmitters (descending modulation) and two of these are particularly important in reducing or modulating the pain experience: **serotonin** and **noradrenalin**. They are both able to inhibit the production of substance P and therefore reduce the pain response by damping down the inflammatory process.

A further group of chemicals produced that modulate the pain experience, by descending mechanisms, are the **endogenous opioids**. Endorphins were named by combining the words endogenous (produced within the body) and morphine. These opioids act directly on the receptors in the central nervous system, very similarly to the way manufactured opioids such as morphine do. Three have been identified:

- Endorphins
- Enkephalins
- Dynorphins

This discovery was confirmed when their action was blocked by the morphine antagonist naloxone. The latter is used in clinical practice as an antidote to the unwanted side effects of an opioid,

---

Case study

Peter is a 27 year old soldier who has been on active duty in the Middle East for the past two months. The situation has been highly dangerous and he has lost several colleagues in combat. Today his team found themselves in a terribly dangerous position, cut off from their main patrol with little support available. Peter faced possible death and knew it was highly unlikely that he would survive. A mortar attack made a direct hit and Peter had his right leg blown off. In the ensuing chaos he realised he had survived and additional troops had managed to get through and rescue them. At the Red Cross camp he felt little pain but an overwhelming sense of relief. He was alive and would soon be going home.

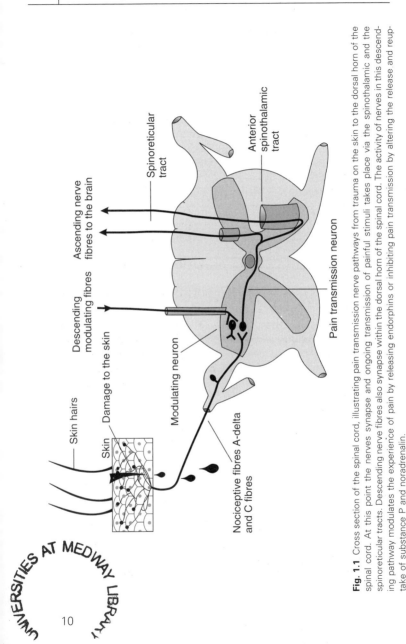

Fig. 1.1 Cross section of the spinal cord, illustrating pain transmission nerve pathways from trauma on the skin to the dorsal horn of the spinal cord. At this point the nerves synapse and ongoing transmission of painful stimuli takes place via the spinothalamic and the spinoreticular tracts. Descending nerve fibres also synapse within the dorsal horn of the spinal cord. The activity of nerves in this descending pathway modulates the experience of pain by releasing endorphins or inhibiting pain transmission by altering the release and reuptake of substance P and noradrenalin.

such as respiratory depression or possible overdose. The case study of Peter demonstrates the power of descending modulation. This modulation could be a response to the strong emotions felt at the time, a phenomenon observed by Beecher during the Second World War (Beecher 1959).

Principal spinal cord and brain anatomy associated with the transmission and experience of pain

- Dorsal root ganglia are located in the area outside the spinal cord where primary afferent nerves have their cell bodies.
- The dorsal horn is the part of the spinal cord where pain-transmitting nerve fibres synapse for the first time or pass on their messages to second order neurons.
- Substantia gelatinosa is a specific area within the dorsal horn of the spinal cord where much of the C fibre synaptic activity takes place.
- The spinothalamic tract transmits information principally to the thalamus.
- The spinoreticular tract transmits principally to the reticular formation.
- The reticular formation, brainstem raphe and hypothalamus are the first areas of the brain where further synaptic activity takes place. These areas are a source of modulation, sympathetic and parasympathetic response and it is probably at this point that pain memory and previous experience help to impact on pain perception and response.
- The thalamus is an area within the brain where sensory and motor information is processed before being relayed to the cerebral cortex or 'thinking' part of the brain. In terms of nociception the thalamus is the brain's 'hot spot'.
- The limbic system, responsible for our emotions, appears to be the principal anatomical area in the brain that responds to painful stimuli with aversive behaviour. The area is closely linked to the hypothalamus, which is responsible for producing the responses to emotional input, including the sympathetic and parasympathetic activity associated with pain.
- The somatosensory cortex is where pain gets very complex as no one area appears to process pain. The brain is interconnected with neurons that all signal to each other; hence pain

is such an individual experience based on each of us having a unique genetic and emotional makeup, history, culture, upbringing and personal view of pain and suffering.

- Periaqueductal grey matter surrounds the cerebral aqueduct in the mid brain. Periaqueductal grey matter contains connections with all levels of the nervous system and therefore plays a vital role in integration through its influence on pain processing, behaviour, response and the autonomic and motor systems. When electrically stimulated in the laboratory setting, subjects report feelings of unpleasantness, fear and sometimes even intense dread – it is a very unpopular experiment!

Figure 1.2 is an illustration of some of the parts of the brain that are known to be associated with pain perception and modulation.

This brief outline of some of the essential 'anatomy' of pain is a huge oversimplification of what is a very complex and dynamic system. For further reading refer to some of the excellent contemporary books on pain such as *Pain: A Textbook for Therapists* edited by Strong et al. (2002), which also includes some clear diagrams.

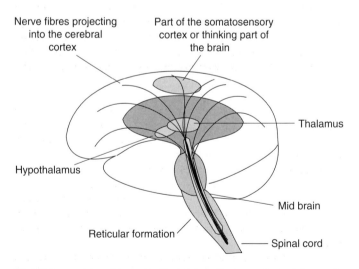

Fig. 1.2 Cross section of the brain, showing the various parts that are important for pain perception and modulation.

> **Box 1.1 Examples of chronic pain**
>
> - Arthritis
> - Central pain (possibly following a stroke)
> - Chronic regional pain syndrome (also called reflex sympathetic dystrophy)
> - Peripheral neuropathies
> - Chronic low back pain
> - Body pain associated with HIV/AIDS

Acute pain can be explained by the gate control theory. However, it is not a panacea for all and there continue to be anomalies and gaps in our knowledge. Much of this is explored in the next section as we expand on chronic pain.

CHRONIC PAIN AND BEYOND

Unlike the acute short-term pain associated with a particular event, such as hitting your finger with a hammer, chronic pain can be viewed as a disorder of the nervous system that persists for months or years and cannot be fully relieved by standard pain medications (Box 1.1). Chronic pain also may cause a problem called **allodynia**, in which people experience pain from stimuli that are not normally painful, such as a light touch or a breeze, or pain in places other than the area that is stimulated. It is often associated with anxiety, depression and interference with social activities.

Recent studies have suggested that the brain not only receives pain signals from the spinal cord but also undergoes changes in neuronal connections that may permanently strengthen its reactions to those signals. Researchers believe these changes are key to the development of chronic pain.

The gate control theory has not explained all we see in people experiencing pain. Indeed it has been adapted and added to over the years. Melzack (1993) has continued to develop pain theory and, working with paraplegics and people suffering phantom limb pain, has started to use the term '**neuromatrix**' to explain their pain.

Millions of nerve impulses hit the nervous system each moment and therefore it is essential for the sense of body to be maintained. Details from these inputs are integrated into the neuromatrix as they arrive, allowing for continual revision, where inputs are analysed and synthesised to produce appropriate responses. From this understanding it can be inferred that commands originating in the brain may actually produce experiences (rather than input from the periphery, associated with acute pain). This may explain why amputees suffer genuine fatigue from the experience of persistent bicycling movements, or relate the feeling of pain from clenching an imaginary fist. The neuromatrix is a more dynamic explanation that accommodates new knowledge to explain how exposure to severe pain has actually changed the infrastructure, at a molecular level, of our own neural pathways. In fact, considerable work has been done using computerised topography to illustrate which regions of the brain are involved (Derbyshire 2000). The neuromatrix explains how:

- Pain is a subjective and personal experience
- It involves many central regions of the brain
- It can be generated from within the brain
- Previous pain experiences can affect future pain experiences

Psychosocial implications of chronic pain

How individuals respond to pain has been suggested as more important than knowledge of physical treatments in individuals with chronic pain (Main & Spanswick 2000). An understanding of the psychosocial factors that may exert such an impact is vital if the care and pain management strategies offered to chronic pain sufferers are to reflect the latest discoveries in the field of science and human behaviour.

Case study

Audrey has experienced severe back pain for the past six years. She stopped working in a local garden centre and now spends most of her time sitting or lying on the sofa watching daytime TV. She has put on 6 kg during the past two years and no longer enjoys seeing her friends or going out. Her husband does as much as he can for her but feels helpless. Sleep is now difficult at night so she dozes when she can in the day.

You may see patients who have become extremely disabled and experience severe intractable pain when identifiable pathology appears to be relatively mild. Other individuals with a similar complaint may report pain but do not develop the same levels of disability. In fact some may appear to maintain a reasonable quality of life despite reporting pain intensity that is severe and prolonged. There is now good evidence that quality of life for patients with chronic pain is more associated with beliefs about pain than with pain intensity (Lame et al. 2004). Throughout the following chapters we will try to use case studies to illustrate the complex interplay of physiology, psychology and the relationship between body and mind in the management of pain.

Assessment and evaluation

Pain assessment is the cornerstone to effective management and there are now a wide variety of tools that help us to assess and record pain and evaluate the interventions used to improve pain control. In subsequent chapters we will be looking at various assessment tools in more detail and applying them to a variety of pain experiences within particular patient groups. To measure the intensity of pain one-dimensional tools are often used. One-dimensional tools only enable you to record pain intensity. Examples of these are the visual analogue scale, the numerical rating scale and the verbal rating scale.

The visual analogue scale is usually a scale of 10 cm (100 mm), which enables the patient's rating of his or her pain to be measured (Fig. 1.3). The scale especially means that small variations in perceived pain intensity may be documented, which is particularly useful for a research study. Some patients find it easier to choose a word (see Fig. 1.4 – the verbal rating scale) or a number (see Fig. 1.5 – the numerical rating scale) to describe their pain.

However, for pain that is chronic, complex or impacting on quality of life many more factors will need to be assessed apart from simply pain intensity and possibly location of the pain or pains. This is particularly important during the first encounter with patients as it establishes that their pain is important and captures baseline data. Multidimensional pain tools often enable the physical and psychosocial impact of the experience of pain to be recorded. Such a pain tool would be helpful for Audrey's pain

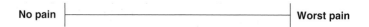

No pain |————————————————————————————————| **Worst pain**

Fig. 1.3 The visual analogue scale (VAS).

None	Mild	Moderate	Severe	Excruciating

Fig. 1.4 The verbal rating scale.

1	2	3	4	5

Fig. 1.5 The numerical rating scale.

described in the previous case study. Figure 1.6 is an example of the short form Brief Pain Inventory which is often used in specialist pain clinics (Cleeland & Ryan 1994).

THERAPEUTIC MANAGEMENT OF PAIN

The principles of pain management underpin all approaches to this unpleasant experience. Effective management of the patient's pain must reflect the multidimensional approaches described in this chapter. The following chapters explore in greater detail the management strategies employed in specific pain situations. It is important to emphasise that no one intervention is sufficient to manage pain if we are to exploit the multidimensional understanding of pain (Table 1.3).

SUMMARY

Understanding the mechanisms responsible for the experience of pain provides us with an excellent base for assessment and treatment. Pain can be viewed as a multidimensional experience with a sensory, cognitive and emotional component. Understanding the neural mechanisms informs the management of pain. Nurses are in a pivotal position to use this knowledge to assess pain and identify how each component of the pain experience can be exploited, using evidence, where available, to bring the patient maximal benefit.

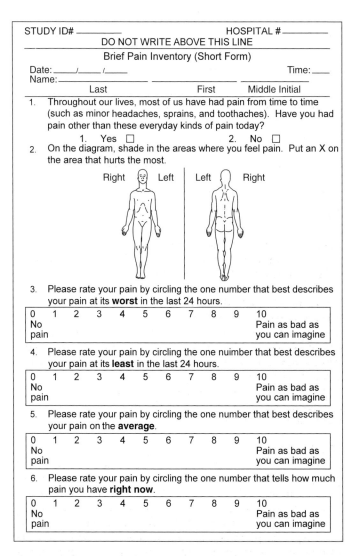

STUDY ID# _____   HOSPITAL # _____
DO NOT WRITE ABOVE THIS LINE

Brief Pain Inventory (Short Form)

Date: ____/____/____   Time: ____
Name: _____   _____   _____
       Last   First   Middle Initial

1. Throughout our lives, most of us have had pain from time to time (such as minor headaches, sprains, and toothaches). Have you had pain other than these everyday kinds of pain today?

      1. Yes ☐   2. No ☐

2. On the diagram, shade in the areas where you feel pain. Put an X on the area that hurts the most.

Right   Left | Left   Right

3. Please rate your pain by circling the one number that best describes your pain at its **worst** in the last 24 hours.

0	1	2	3	4	5	6	7	8	9	10
No pain										Pain as bad as you can imagine

4. Please rate your pain by circling the one nuimber that best describes your pain at its **least** in the last 24 hours.

0	1	2	3	4	5	6	7	8	9	10
No pain										Pain as bad as you can imagine

5. Please rate your pain by circling the one number that best describes your pain on the **average**.

0	1	2	3	4	5	6	7	8	9	10
No pain										Pain as bad as you can imagine

6. Please rate your pain by circling the one number that tells how much pain you have **right now**.

0	1	2	3	4	5	6	7	8	9	10
No pain										Pain as bad as you can imagine

Fig. 1.6 Brief Pain Inventory (short form). (Reproduced with kind permission of Prof Charles S. Cleeland. Available at www.ohsu.edu.ahec.pain.paininventory.pdf.)

Cont.

Fig. 1.6 *Continued.*

---

7. What treatments or medications are you receiving for your pain?

_____

8. In the last 24 hours, how much relief have pain treatments or medications provided? Please circle the one percentage that most shows how much **relief** you have received.

0%	10%	20%	30%	40%	50%	60%	70%	80%	90%	100%
No relief										Complete relief

9. Circle the one number that describes how, during the past 24 hours, pain has interfered with your:

A. General activity

0	1	2	3	4	5	6	7	8	9	10
Does not interfere										Completely interferes

B. Mood

0	1	2	3	4	5	6	7	8	9	10
Does not interfere										Completely interferes

C. Walking ability

0	1	2	3	4	5	6	7	8	9	10
Does not interfere										Completely interferes

D. Normal work (includes both work outside the home and housework)

0	1	2	3	4	5	6	7	8	9	10
Does not interfere										Completely interferes

E. Relations with other people

0	1	2	3	4	5	6	7	8	9	10
Does not interfere										Completely interferes

F. Sleep

0	1	2	3	4	5	6	7	8	9	10
Does not interfere										Completely interferes

G. Enjoyment of life

0	1	2	3	4	5	6	7	8	9	10
Does not interfere										Completely interferes

Table 1.3 The multidimensional components of pain and associated management strategies.

Experiencing pain – multidimensional components	Management strategies

Sensory factors
• Injury and tissue damage
	• Pharmacological strategies
	  ○ Opioids (such as morphine), which bind to receptors in the CNS and alter the perception of pain
	  ○ Non-steroidal anti-inflammatory drugs (NSAIDs), paracetamol and aspirin
	  ○ Anti-epileptic drugs, antidepressants and local anaesthetics
	• Cutaneous stimulation, e.g. transcutaneous electrical nerve stimulation, massage, acupuncture, heat or cold therapies
	• Comfort strategies – positioning, warmth

Cognitive factors • Being able to focus on the pain (night) • No outside interests/distractions • Worrying about the pain	• Distraction – chatting, imagery, television, radio • Skilled companionship – being with the patient, listening to his or her pain experience • Patient and family education about pain • Sensory input – music, aromatherapy
Emotional factors • Depression • Anxiety • Stress • Frustration • Hopelessness	• Self-help strategies – biofeedback • Relaxation strategies • Rehabilitation and re-mobilisation strategies, exercise

REFERENCES

Beecher, H.K. (1959) *Measurement of Subjective Responses: Quantitative Effects of Drugs.* Oxford University Press, New York.

Cleeland, C.S. & Ryan, K.M. (1994) Pain assessment: global use of the Brief Pain Inventory. *Annals of the Academy of Medicine* **23** (2), 129–138.

Derbyshire, S. (2000) Exploring the pain neuromatrix. *Current Review of Pain* **4**, 467–477.

International Association for the Study of Pain (1986) Classification of chronic pain. Descriptions of chronic pain syndromes and definitions of pain terms. *Pain* (Suppl. 3), S1–S226.

Lame, I.E., Peters, M.L., Vlaeyen, J.W. et al. (2004) Quality of life in chronic pain is more associated with beliefs about pain, than with pain intensity. *European Journal of Pain* **9**, 15–24.

Main, C.J. & Spanswick, C.C. (2000) *Pain Management: An Interdisciplinary Approach.* Churchill Livingstone, London.

McCaffery, M. (1968) *Nursing Practice Theories Related to Cognition, Bodily Pain and Non-Environment Interactions.* University of California, Los Angeles.

Melzack, R. (1993) Pain: past, present and future. *Canadian Journal of Experimental Psychology* **47** (4), 615–629.

Strong, J., Unruh, A.M., Wright, A. & Baxter, G.D. (eds) (2002) *Pain: A Textbook for Therapists.* Churchill Livingstone, London.

Types of Pain and Basic Strategies for Pain Management

2

INTRODUCTION

This chapter expands on the previous chapter that described the theories and mechanisms of pain and explores in more depth the various types of pain and the potential impact pain has on an individual. It also begins to describe some of the strategies used for pain management. Examples of further reading resources, where available, are given in order to help inform clinical practice. Nurses are often with the patient in pain more than any other member of the health care team and are well placed to accurately assess pain and ensure that interventions reflect the multidimensional nature of the pain experience.

LEARNING OBJECTIVES

❑ To identify the various types of pain
❑ To briefly discuss the possible causes of a range of painful conditions
❑ To outline the basic principles of pain management

DIFFERENT TYPES OF PAIN

Acute pain

This term refers to pain of limited duration that is related to a specific event or onset of illness. It is associated with hyperactivity within the autonomic nervous system and will usually respond well to analgesia. If pain is severe, then exploiting our knowledge of pain pathways, in combination with analgesia that blocks nerve impulses (local anaesthetics), modifies the impact on the central nervous system (opioids) and reduces the inflammatory response (non-steroidal anti-inflammatory drugs), will usually produce excellent pain control. Acute pain should be easy to manage, but optimising pain control strategies remains problematic. Some of the barriers that appear to impact on effective pain management are explored in Chapter 8.

Chronic pain

This describes pain that has usually lasted weeks or more or is associated with a pathological process that is ongoing or degenerative. This pain is much more difficult to treat as changes take place within the peripheral and central nervous system, which may completely alter the choices of therapy available to control it. Continuous, enduring pain will have a considerable emotional and social impact. When analgesia does not work and pain fails to respond to the usual therapies, the psychosocial consequences can be considerable. The psychosocial impacts are not necessarily confined to the sufferer; frequently his or her family and friends will be affected if pain continues indefinitely. When pain becomes severe and intractable there may ultimately be a negative impact on the economy and society in general as sufferers withdraw from social interaction and become economically inactive, destined to live an unproductive and unfulfilling life on incapacity benefit.

Somatic pain

Somatic pain describes pain confined to the body wall or musculoskeletal system. If skin or subcutaneous tissue is also involved then it is sometimes referred to as superficial somatic or cutaneous pain. Pain is usually easy to locate and can be increased by activity or direct contact. Damage to tissue, muscle and bone will normally repair within 6–8 weeks.

Visceral pain

Visceral pain is felt differently to pain originating from muscle, skin, bone or the connective tissue of the body wall. Visceral pain only originates from internal organs such as the stomach, uterus, bowel or gall bladder. It is dull, diffused, initially difficult to locate and is often accompanied by a sickening feeling. The lack of the pain-sensitive nerve fibres that proliferate within peripheral tissues such as the skin means that cutting, burning or pinching internal organs is not perceived as pain. However, the following can lead to extreme discomfort and distress, with a magnified autonomic response:

- Distension
- Spasm
- Twisting
- Chemical irritation (such as food poisoning)
- Inflammation
- Ischaemia often felt secondary to the other causes

Nociceptive pain

Nociceptive pain is the term used to describe acute pain associated with the inflammatory and biological processes described in Chapter 1.

Neuropathic pain

Neuropathic pain describes pain resulting from current or past damage to peripheral and or central nerves. See Fig. 2.1 for possible examples of nerve damage. The pain may come from within the nervous system itself, rather than be generated as a result of nociception. Initial nociception may leave an imprint on the central nervous system that results in pain failing to fade away as the tissues heal. Nerves may become damaged because they were torn, severed or compressed during trauma, or may be cut during surgery or amputation. A metabolic disorder such as diabetes or a virus such as herpes may also have damaging consequences. Diseases such as multiple sclerosis or endometriosis may cause nerve disruption or scarring, leading to the potential for long-term neuropathic or neurogenic pain. Several types of neuropathic pain may develop such as the following:

- Complex regional pain syndrome 1, previously known as reflex sympathetic dystrophy (this does not involve a specific nerve lesion at the start)
- Complex regional pain syndrome 2, previously known as causalgia (this begins with a nerve injury)
- Scar pain which may involve entrapment of specific nerves or may eventually be found to be a form of complex regional pain syndrome
- Central pain which may develop when damage has occurred to the central nervous system, thalamus or spinal cord possibly as a result of a stroke

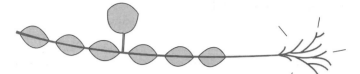

(a) A cut nerve begins to regenerate, the sprouts are mechanically sensitive and activated by sympathetic α-adrenergic stimulation

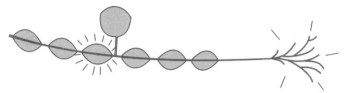

(b) A second site of activity, stimulated by α-adrenergic neurotransmitters, can develop near the dorsal root ganglion

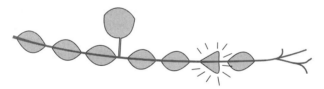

(c) A third site of pain transmission can develop following a small area of demylination on a primary afferent which can lead to ectopic impulse generation

Fig. 2.1 Some of the possible causes of the development of neuropathic pain syndromes.

- Deafferentation pain which occurs when nerves have been torn away as may happen with a brachial plexus avulsion
- Peripheral neuropathies which occur when nerves have been damaged or have died. Cutting and tearing, ischaemia, compression, toxicity, etc. may cause this damage
- Phantom limb pain which may be due to neuroma formation or alterations in processing within the central nervous system

CAUSES OF ACUTE PAIN

Surgery

Surgery inevitably causes damage to soft tissues, nerves and possibly bone. Incisions through large muscles may be particularly painful as well as procedures that involve bone harvesting for grafts or remodelling. No two people will experience a surgical procedure in the same way, but as you would expect, the larger the wound, the greater the potential for pain. Considerable pain is usually associated with incisions involving the upper abdomen and chest wall. A number of procedures can now be undertaken laparoscopically and the avoidance of muscle damage and the minimal invasion of body cavities can greatly reduce the need for prolonged analgesia.

Trauma

Trauma may result in peripheral pain confined to skin and subcutaneous tissues or may include musculoskeletal injury resulting in pain secondary to sprains or strains, tearing or crushing injuries. Any trauma may cause haematoma formation, acute inflammation, swelling and potentially secondary infection.

Disease

Many disease processes or metabolic disorders cause pain. Often it is pain that first leads to patients seeking medical help. Any hollow organ that has a blockage or is becoming inflamed will become acutely tender. A disease process that is swelling and distorting bone will cause pain from the periosteum which is richly innervated, as well as from bone itself as nerve endings grow into the 'hot spots' of inflammation. Alterations in musculoskeletal function can lead to muscle spasm, aching joints and eventually the risk of chronic pain from deconditioning as function and mobility are reduced or lost. Conditions such as osteoporosis may result in breaks to bone that has been stripped of its strength and integrity. Nerves become damaged from metabolic disorders such as diabetes or viral infections such as shingles and AIDS. All of these processes carry the risk that, if left untreated, the initial acutely painful experience may develop into chronic and intractable pain as hyperactivity in any part of the nervous system fails to revert to its original quiescent state.

CAUSES OF CHRONIC PAIN

Most pain is self-limiting, usually related to an acute event and gradually resolves over time. However, unfortunately that is not always the case. For some people the underlying cause may be relatively easy to understand, as in the case of an inflammatory condition such as rheumatoid arthritis or as a result of ischaemia associated with peripheral vascular disease. They are referred to as having chronic pain but may in fact have long periods when they are pain free or pain is only brought on by activity. However, for many chronic pain sufferers the exact cause of ongoing pain may not be so straightforward. Even though science is now making substantial breakthroughs in helping us understand how some pain syndromes may develop, many remain something of an enigma, with allusive pathology to account for the pain.

Chronic neuropathic pain

Neuropathic pain can develop rapidly in the acute phase of any insult, particularly when a major nerve or plexus is damaged, e.g. phantom limb pain. However, neuropathic pain does not just develop following damage to major nerve structures; minor damage or disease may leave nerve fibres trying to regenerate with abnormal connections to the sympathetic nervous system. Nerves may have bits of their myelin sheath missing, or following trans-section may be regenerating bundles of nervelets rather than a single nerve fibre (see Fig. 2.1). Any of these factors may lead to nerves misfiring or developing abnormal function with scrambled messages and excessive neurological chatter.

This can be perplexing for patients and health care professionals, as tissue might look healthy but pain is evident. You cannot scan, X-ray or undertake nerve conduction studies to discover the cause and patients often say they feel their pain is not believed (Clarke & Iphofen 2005). This is a typical feature of neuropathic pain, where you may only have the clinical description from the patient to go on and no obvious pathology or cause.

Chronic musculoskeletal pain

Chronic musculoskeletal pain describes any long-standing pain that is attributed to muscle, bone, fascia, ligaments, tendons, joints, etc. and will present clinically with a variety of underlying features. Commonly it is associated with diseases such as arthritis or age-related degeneration of joints. In some instances it may develop as a disuse syndrome where acute pain has led to inactivity (Nederhand et al. 2003). Like the development of any complex pain it is better described within the biopsychosocial rather than the biomedical model (Melzack 1999).

Chronic visceral pain

Chronic visceral pain remains poorly understood, although some conditions are linked to inflammatory changes of unknown etiology, especially some of the urogenital and pelvic pain syndromes such as:

- Loin pain/haematuria syndrome
- Interstitial cystitis
- Irritable bowel syndrome
- Prostatodynia (prostatitis)
- Vulvular vestibulitis

Pain may result from a complex mix of functional disorder, neurogenic dysfunction, genetic predisposition, stress or an ongoing disease process such as chronic endometriosis or pancreatitis. It may also be present when no disease process can be identified such as the experience of chronic chest pain in patients with angiographically normal coronary arteries.

PSYCHOSOCIAL IMPACTS OF PAIN

Pain is unique to each of us, but how our immediate family and friends respond to our reports of pain may alter our behaviour, especially during our formative years. Was little made of our injuries as we were told not to fuss, or did we grow up in a family where every scratch and scrape was accompanied by great drama and distress? Not only is our response and the response of those around us significant, there is now evidence that our genetic makeup also has some bearing on the severity of any pain we experience (Buskila et al. 2005). The impact of culture and society's expectations help influence our behaviour to be vocal and expressive or reserved and quietly tolerant (Brand & Yancy 1993). In 1952 Zborowski undertook the first major studies into cultural differences in the way people respond to pain. Culture may well be an important consideration affecting the way pain and illness are expressed through learned behaviour patterns (Bernstein & Pachter 1993).

GENDER INFLUENCES

The sexes have even been subjected to experimental pain in order to study differences in their responses and many of these studies have been published (Mitchell et al. 2004). Unruh (1996, 1997), Unruh & Campbell (1999), Unruh & McGrath (2000) and Unruh et al. (1999) have published extensively on the subject of gender and pain. More recently there have been studies looking at gender and specific types of pain such as the vascular pain of heart disease (Kimble et al. 2003) and pain related to osteoarthritis (Keefe et al. 2004).

Attitudes to pain and beliefs and appraisal concerning pain have a strong influence on how each of us perceives pain (Unruh et al. 1999). As Morris (1991, p. 29) puts it, 'we experience pain only and entirely as we interpret it'. It is unique to each individual. Each chapter will therefore include reference to psychological and social dimensions of the pain experience as well as some of the biological mechanisms that are thought to imprint a pain memory on our central nervous systems.

Society, culture, genetics and our upbringing have an impact on the pain we experience, and initial biological insults can result in a wide range of pains. The causes of pain will influence its management; therefore each chapter will describe the various organic causes that may initiate pain especially pertaining to particular age groups. Pain may be acute or chronic, visceral or somatic, nociceptive or neuropathic or a combination of all of these. There are of course instances where people feel pain and no reason for this can be found and we include these situations too.

STRATEGIES TO MANAGE PAIN

Specific strategies for managing pain will be covered in more detail within each chapter, giving the potential problems associated with various drugs particularly when given to vulnerable people such as the very young, the very elderly or the particularly ill patient.

Pharmacological strategies

Although research into pain management has expanded rapidly, many of the drugs we use to treat pain have been around a very long time. The expansion in choice is often down to the development of synthetic and semisynthetic compounds of some tried and tested analgesics that have been used for hundreds of years. One of the most important factors influencing the decision to prescribe or administer a drug is the evidence available concerning its effectiveness and the risks associated with its use.

Evidence-based practice

For the best evidence on which analgesics are effective and which are not, *Bandolier*, an electronic journal, helps to provide a clinical bottom line by summarising grade 1 evidence from randomised controlled trials (see www.jr2.ox.ac.uk/bandolier). They give us NNTs, which stands for 'numbers needed to treat'. Essentially this number represents the number of people who have to receive a particular analgesic at a particular strength for just one of them to achieve a 50% reduction in the perceived intensity of their pain that was not achieved by a placebo. Within these trials, patients in pain are randomised to receive either the active analgesic or a placebo and their pain score using a numerical rating is recorded. We know that pain can often respond very well for a short time to a placebo, although this mechanism is not fully understood. Because of the potentially powerful placebo response sometimes obtainable in the presence of very real nociceptive pain, a calculation is made to remove this response from the final equation. What that means is the lower the NNT, the more effective the drug (Box 2.1).

Box 2.1 Numbers needed to treat (NNTs)

For the treatment of acute pain – ibuprofen 400 mg has an NNT of 2.4 and paracetamol 1 g has an NNT of 3.8. Many people think codeine 60 mg is a much stronger analgesic and yet it has an NNT of 16.7 and is often associated with unwanted side effects such as constipation.

However, the data available to us, even when they represent grade 1 evidence based on meta-analysis of multiple good quality randomised controlled trials, always have to be put into the context of both the patients and their clinician experiences. The most effective drugs are of no use if patients just do not like them or resist taking them because of unpleasant side effects or powerful myths and misconceptions surrounding their use. The development of 'clinical bottom lines' on drug efficacy may not always capture the fact that patients may be lost to a trial simply because they did not like the drug. Critics of NNTs observe that these trials often exclude older people with several diseases and that the samples often include all surgical patients rather than a homogenous group.

Data taken from the Oxford League Table of Analgesic Efficacy within *Bandolier* are an extremely valuable resource (www.jr2.ox.ac.uk/bandolier). The following is a brief synopsis of some of the key highlights:

- The efficacy of weak opioids on their own appears to be very poor, with codeine 60 mg representing the highest NNT and therefore the least effective analgesic at 16.7.
- The NSAIDs and Cox-2s perform well.
- A previously very popular analgesic in the community, two tablets of co-proxamal representing 65 mg of dextropropoxyphene combined with 650 mg of paracetamol produces an NNT of 4.4, but this is outperformed by paracetamol 1,000 mg alone at 3.8, and co-proxamal has now finally been withdrawn.
- Tramadol 100 mg is also currently outperformed by paracetamol 1 g with an NNT of 4.8 but results in a significantly higher incidence of nausea and vomiting compared to placebo.

With our current knowledge of the lack of efficacy of codeine, its use today may well be questioned (Sachs 2005). As an antitussive agent or a treatment for diarrhoea it may have a place, but as an analgesic even when combined with paracetamol, is it worth the side effects? Unfortunately there are no trials currently available that provide us with an NNT for paracetamol combined with a low dose of oral morphine, the gold standard opioid (British National Formulary 2004). However, a trial of just paracetamol 500 mg with oxycodone (a strong opioid) 5 mg matches the paracetamol 1,000 mg with codeine 60 mg NNT of 2.2. The dose of the strong opioid is very small and may well result in fewer side effects such as nausea, sedation, hallucination or constipation.

Codeine is a pro-drug that has to bioconvert to exert its action. Studies since the late 1970s have confirmed that codeine metabolises to norcodeine and morphine. However, further work during the 1990s on genetic variation and the wide range of codeine activity suggested that some individuals lack the ability to bioconvert codeine to morphine and somewhere between 7 and 10% of the Caucasian population may experience side effects but little in the way of analgesia.

The constipating effects of codeine are well documented and when used long term in the elderly can cause significant distress. Elderly patients may even face the indignity of manual removal of faeces possibly as a direct result of high dose codeine use.

Further anomalies surrounding the NNTs for weak opioid/paracetamol combinations are as follows:

- When codeine 60 mg is added to just paracetamol 650 mg the NNT is 4.2, but this is outperformed by paracetamol 1 g on its own.
- When codeine 60 mg is added to aspirin 650 mg (NNT of 4.4), the NNT actually increases to a worse figure of 5.3.

Paracetamol

This effective drug is available as an intravenous (IV) preparation, in tablet and capsule format, as a liquid or suppository. Paracetamol has analgesic and antipyretic properties with effects comparable to those of aspirin, but it is not an anti-inflammatory drug. Although the mechanisms of paracetamol are not fully understood it is known to be a weak inhibitor of peripheral Cox-1 and -2, the enzymes responsible for synthesising prostaglandins. Paracetamol appears to inhibit prostaglandin biosynthesis in the central nervous system but not in the peripheral tissues (Greenstein 2004), and when given IV may not display the ceiling effect reported with the oral preparation but a dose-dependent increase in peak plasma concentration (Piguet et al. 1998). There are virtually no groups of people who should not take it and interactions with other treatments are rare; however, caution is always advised if a patient has liver disease. At the recommended dosage there are few side effects. Paracetamol is particularly useful as it can be taken by patients sensitive to aspirin and is well tolerated by previous sufferers of peptic ulcer disease. Some newer information suggests there may be a problem with a small percentage of asthmatic patients, but further research is needed.

Non-steroidal anti-inflammatory drugs (NSAIDs)

Some forms of NSAIDs are available in an IV/IM preparation, tablets, capsules, liquid, sublingual or suppository form. Formulated for topical application as creams, sprays or gels, NSAIDs appear to avoid the risk of serious side effects whilst still providing analgesia for certain conditions (Vaile & Davis 1998). These drugs have analgesic, anti-inflammatory and antipyretic properties, but the degree to which various drugs are effective may vary considerably. They are thought to act by inhibiting the biosynthesis of prostaglandins by inhibition of cyclo-oxygenase (Cox) enzymes. They may also act centrally to block some of the components of neurological 'wind up' which leads to an augmented response and heightened sensitivity to pain. Unfortunately, although very effective, they are associated with several adverse side effects particularly when taken regularly over a period of time or when taken by the elderly. Significant problems with NSAIDs are associated with acid secretions and inhibition of the production of the protective layer of mucous within the gastrointestinal tract, leading to damage that may be symptom free (Davis 1999). NSAIDs may also reduce renal blood flow and urine formation, with high doses leading to nephropathy and renal failure especially in the elderly or poorly hydrated patients (Jordan & White 2001). There is now also thought to be a risk of cardiovascular adverse effects, especially in patients with a pre-existing heart condition. NSAIDs can also be problematic for a small percentage of asthma sufferers.

Cox-2s

Some forms of Cox-2s are available IV or IM and there are also tablets and capsules. Like NSAIDs they are very effective analgesics that were originally developed to provide the benefits of NSAIDs but without the gastrointestinal toxicity risk. Unfortunately problems have been established for patients with cardiovascular disease and research is ongoing to establish their place and whether the problems are associated with specific Cox-2s or all in the class.

Opioids

These drugs are in fact extremely safe when used appropriately at the correct dose. The word opioid incorporates both weak and strong preparations.

Weak opioids

As stated earlier these include preparations such as codeine and dihydrocodeine which on their own provide only limited pain relief. They should not continue to be used if they do not prove effective, but frequently patients will be prescribed a range of weak opioids rather than progressing up the 'analgesic ladder' to a stronger opioid. Closer analysis of the barriers to opioid prescribing will be covered in the Chapter 8. Unlike morphine, weak opioids also appear to have a ceiling effect so increasing dosages above the normally prescribed range will not improve pain relief.

Morphine

Drugs such as morphine have been around for a very long time and their adverse side effect profile is well established. Opioids are vital for the treatment of moderate to severe acute pain usually as part of a multimodal regime. Their use in chronic non-malignant pain is somewhat more controversial. For excellent guidance the British Pain Society provides information for prescribers and patients which is downloadable from their website (www.britishpainsociety.org).

Pethidine

Pethidine is a questionable analgesic (McCaffery & Pasero 1999). It is extremely short acting, may give the promise of excellent pain control especially with some visceral pains, but is toxic in moderate to large doses. There are now much better alternatives around, although pethidine still remains popular in some obstetric units and is sometimes given when analgesia will only be required for a brief period of time.

Oxycodone and hydromorphone
These are useful opioids, with oxycodone appearing to have fewer adverse side effects than morphine (Kalso et al. 1991).

Methadone
Methadone can be quite difficult to titrate due to its very long half-life but has a place when prescribed by experts.

Fentanyl
Short-acting opioids such as IV fentanyl can be useful for brief pain or procedures. In a patch[1] formulation fentanyl can be effective for some chronic non-malignant as well as malignant pain and their replacement every three days can be useful when compliance or the oral route is problematic.

Tramadol
Tramadol is often referred to as an opioid but is only very weakly active at the mu receptor. Adverse effects include nausea in up to 35% of postoperative patients along with other opioid-type side effects such as dizziness, sedation and headache, although the risk of respiratory depression is greatly reduced (Vickers et al. 1992). This drug also has an influence on the noradrenalin and serotonin pathways and may find a place in the short-term treatment of subacute and chronic pains.

Tricyclic antidepressants
Tricyclic antidepressants inhibit the re-uptake of noradrenalin and serotonin, neurotransmitters that are thought to be involved in the descending pain inhibitory pathways that modulate pain. Amitriptyline is usually the first line treatment for pain that is becoming chronic, especially when sleep quality is being impaired. Unfortunately amitriptyline has an unpleasant side effect profile and above a very low dose is often poorly tolerated especially by the elderly.

---

[1] Patches are also available containing buprenorphine and these are sometimes used as an alternative to the fentanyl patch.

Anticonvulsants

Anticonvulsants are regarded as effective for the treatment of neuropathic pain and may be used instead of or as well as low dose tricyclic antidepressants. They are thought to work by stabilising neuronal membranes, making them less likely to fire ectopically or erratically. Gabapentin may also inhibit nociceptive transmission in the central nervous system and its role as part of a multimodal strategy for perioperative pain is being investigated (Gilron 2002). In some countries, gabapentin is beginning to replace amitriptyline as a first line treatment for some neuropathic pain.

NMDA-receptor antagonists

Again these appear to be useful for the management of some chronic neuropathic pain states although the side effects of ketamine, the principal drug currently prescribed, limits its use at present. Ketamine combined with midazolam, a benzodiazepine, appears to provide useful analgesia enhanced by patient amnesia of an unpleasant experience. This can be particularly beneficial when offering conscious sedation as a viable and safe alternative for patients who have to undergo a particularly painful procedure, such as a burns dressing that would previously have required a general anaesthetic (SIGN 2005; Averley et al. 2004).

Local anaesthetics

These are available as topical gels and creams as well as in an injectable format for blocking peripheral nerves and for regional anaesthesia. Common techniques for pain management include brachial plexus, intercostal, ilioinguinal, sciatic and tibial nerve blocks. The quality of the analgesia can be extremely good, with little in the way of systemic side effects although loss of sensation and/or motor block may be problematic. Local anaesthetic patches may well prove to be particularly useful for neuropathic pain that is confined to one specific area and where a patch can be conveniently located.

Inhalational analgesia

Entonox can be very useful for short painful procedures and is probably underutilised, especially in the community (see Fig.

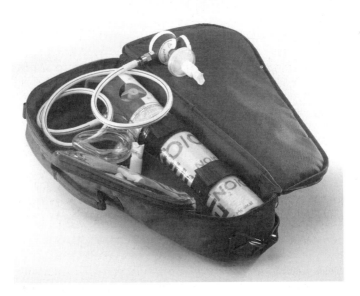

Fig. 2.2 An Entonox cylinder and demand apparatus. (Photograph gratefully received from BOC Ltd.)

2.2). It does not need a prescription as it is very safe when used following training. As well as the more common contraindications such as head injury, pneumothorax or any condition that could cause gas to diffuse into a space causing potentially fatal expansion (Sealey 2002), it should be avoided in the following patients:

- Those with pulmonary oedema, pulmonary hypertension and mitral stenosis
- Those with reduced respiratory drive as it reduces natural ventilatory stimulation
- Pregnant women in the first and second trimester
- Patients requiring more than a short burst of pain relief as bone marrow suppression can occur due to the inactivation of B_{12} from exposures lasting just 2–4 hours

Resources

- Bandolier: www.jr2.ox.ac.uk/bandolier
- Oxford League Table of Analgesic Efficacy: www.jr2.ox.ac.uk/bandolier/booth/painpag/acutrev/analgesics/iftab
- The Medicines and Healthcare Products Regulatory Agency is the government agency responsible for the safety of medicines and medical products. The site gives advice on analgesic options for the treatment of mild to moderate pain in adults and following the proposed withdrawal of co-proxamol. Visit www.mhra.gov.uk and click through to the section on safety information
- The Paracetamol Information Centre: www.pharmweb.net/pwmirror/pwy/paracetamol/pharmwebpic.html
- For more information on problems associated with NSAIDs see the Bandolier section on NSAIDs and adverse effects: www.jr2.ox.ac.uk/bandolier/booth/painpag/nsae/nsae
- The National Prescribing Centre briefing on NSAIDs and gastroprotection: www.npc.co.uk/merec_briefings/2002/briefing_no_20.pdf
- See also Evans (2003) for an article on Entonox in the community for the control of procedural pain

Basic rules for the effective use of analgesia and adjuvants

The golden rule for pain management is to assess current pain or pains experienced and evaluate each strategy used for each and every individual. This is particularly important when pain is going to increase or be caused by the action of health care professionals. It is imperative to act on the evaluation, adjust interventions if necessary and repeat the assessment at regular intervals. If it is appearing unlikely that one strategy will offer adequate analgesia consider increasing dosages if necessary, adding in additional pharmacological strategies and combining these with non-pharmacological therapy. Multimodal therapy using a range of different pharmacological and complementary strategies is usually required for any pain that is becoming severe. Only mild pain will usually respond well to a single strategy such as two paracetamol 500 mg tablets. Do not leave patients having to cope with an analgesic regimen that is either inappropriate or inadequate. Each person will need a regimen individually tailored to his or her needs with strategies in place to counteract any potential side effects. There is no such thing as a one size fits all policy. Some helpful points are as follows:

- In a secondary care environment, such as a hospital/nursing home/residential care, a prescription that includes simple analgesia and/or adjuvants with the option to add in opioids as needed will enable nursing staff to mix and match according to each patient's individual response or medical history.
- Within a primary care setting, the option to titrate strong opioids may be more problematic, but this and the use of adjuvant therapies will be covered in more detail when exploring various scenarios.

Other strategies usually confined to or initiated within secondary care

Patient controlled analgesia pumps
These are programmable portable pumps that can be activated by patients pressing a button (Figs. 2.3 and 2.4). Once activated, small doses of morphine or a similar opioid can be delivered intravenously to enable patients to adjust their own levels of analgesia and balance side effects. The devices are safe as they have a lockout period programmed into them that ensures patients

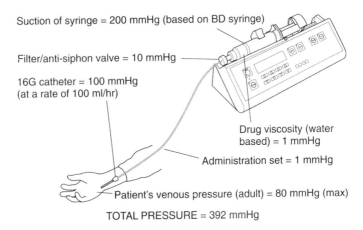

Suction of syringe = 200 mmHg (based on BD syringe)

Filter/anti-siphon valve = 10 mmHg

16G catheter = 100 mmHg
(at a rate of 100 ml/hr)

Drug viscosity (water based) = 1 mmHg

Administration set = 1 mmHg

Patient's venous pressure (adult) = 80 mmHg (max)

TOTAL PRESSURE = 392 mmHg

Fig. 2.3 Example of a patient controlled analgesia pump. (Reproduced with kind permission of Smith Medical Ltd.)

cannot access multiple top-ups and risk overdose. Research and experience over many years suggests that for most adults a bolus dose of 1 mg morphine with a five-minute lockout period provides an effective regime. As with all strong opioids there is a small risk of respiratory depression in the range of 0.2%, which is easily treated with the reversal agent naloxone. This represents less of a risk than is associated with either intermittent IM injections or continuous IV infusions of opioids (Baird & Schug 1996).

Advantages include:

- Patient preference and enhanced pain control
- Individualised administration
- Rapid titration
- Possible beneficial savings in nursing time
- Possible reduced time to discharge

Disadvantages include:

- Potential for infection via cannula
- Requirement for skilled nursing and pharmacy support
- Some patients prefer not to have control
- Expensive pumps and maintenance
- Cost of disposables

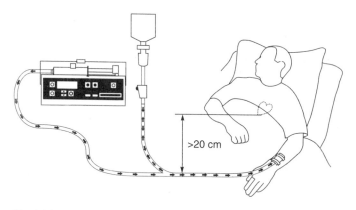

>20 cm

Fig. 2.4 Locating a patient controlled analgesia pump. (Reproduced with kind permission of Smith Medical Ltd.)

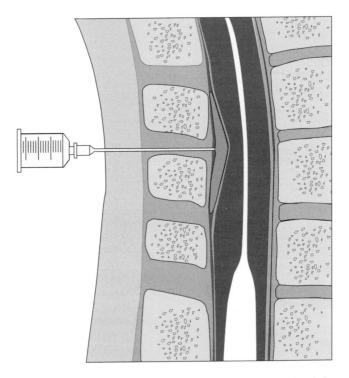

Fig. 2.5 Location of an epidural catheter, which is threaded through a hollow cannula once this has been placed within the epidural space. (Reproduced with kind permission of Smith Medical Ltd.)

Continuous epidural analgesia

This provides analgesia via a small catheter inserted into the epidural space surrounding the spinal cord in the patient's back (Fig. 2.5). It is a particularly useful intervention following major abdominal, thoracic or lower limb surgery or during labour. A continuous infusion of local anaesthetic or more commonly a combination of local anaesthetic and a lipid soluble opioid such as fentanyl or diamorphine are most commonly used.

To undertake the safe placement of this catheter, patients need to be either sitting up with their back and necks curved forward

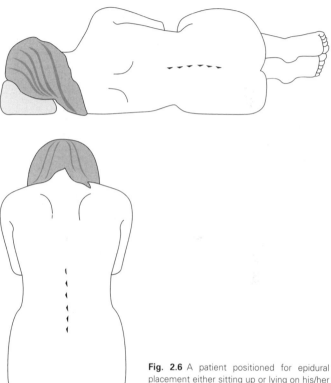

Fig. 2.6 A patient positioned for epidural placement either sitting up or lying on his/her side. (Reproduced with kind permission of Smith Medical Ltd.)

or curled into a ball on their sides to ensure the spaces between the spinal vertebrae are opened up as much as possible. See Fig. 2.6 for illustrations of ideal patient positions.

When it is anticipated that pain may be severe, epidurals can provide extremely good analgesia with the potential to improve outcome through a reduction in morbidity and possibly mortality (Ballantyne et al. 1998). Although requiring close monitoring, patients with an epidural can be effectively nursed in any acute setting following additional education of nursing and medical staff (Richardson 2001). Epidurals are associated with several favourable outcomes:

- Preserved gastrointestinal function and early oral feeding (Lui et al. 1995)
- Reduced incidence of pulmonary infections, atelectasis and hypoxaemia (Ballentyne et al. 1998)
- Reduced stress response and breakdown of body protein and energy sources (Kehlet 1989)
- This may well contribute to a reduction in the risk of immunosuppression with its resulting increased risk of infection (Melzack 1999)
- Reduced incidence of thromboembolic complications (Jorgensen et al. 1991)
- Reduced oxygen requirement of the heart leading to fewer fatal arrhythmias and myocardial infarction following upper abdominal surgery (de Leon-Casasola 1996)

Theoretical disadvantages include the following:

- Tolerance may occur sooner
- Risk of infection
- Risk of haematoma formation close to the spinal cord
- Contraindicated for some patients, e.g. with clotting disorders
- Intravascular migration
- Intradural migration
- Requires special expertise to site
- Requires special monitoring
- Cost of pumps and disposables

Skills and knowledge for managing epidural infusions
Nurses should monitor and document:

- Pain intensity
- Level of sedation
- Degree of motor and sensory blockade
- Vital signs
- The cannula insertion site at frequent intervals but at least daily in patients with no reported symptoms

---

> **Box 2.2 Nurses' knowledge and skills of epidural infusions**
>
> An Australian study involving 153 registered nurses at a large general hospital assessed their knowledge of managing epidural infusions using a survey and simulated clinical scenarios. The findings suggested that nurses had good knowledge levels of pain assessment and sensory blockage but poor knowledge levels of motor blockage assessment and pharmacological side effects. These findings stress the importance of combining education with clinical decision-making skills (Bird & Wallis 2002).

This monitoring should be conducted by nursing staff who have received specific teaching about epidural infusions and the management of these methods, as well as the potential adverse effects (Box 2.2). See Appendix 2.1 for an epidural observation chart.

Spinal analgesia

Spinal or intrathecal analgesia is usually given pre-operatively to provide anaesthesia for surgery and profound pain relief for the immediate postoperative period. This technique may provide analgesia for as long as 12–24 hours (Boezaart et al. 1999) and work is currently taking place to develop even longer lasting local anaesthetic agents. A fine needle is inserted into the cerebrospinal fluid surrounding the spinal cord and usually a combination of heavy local anaesthetic and an opioid such as diamorphine is injected as a single shot rather than as a continuous infusion. This technique is usually used for urological, gynaecological and orthopaedic procedures when patients will be able to rapidly tolerate effective oral analgesia as the local block wears off. Unlike epidural analgesia, patients are usually left with a temporary motor and sensory block, as even small doses of local anaesthetic injected directly onto the spinal cord will affect the nerves below the insertion level.

Non-pharmacological strategies

The most exciting aspect of many of these interventions is that nurses can directly advocate their use without a prescription. One of the central activities of nursing care is to provide comfort and help in the relief of pain. We emphasise the importance of utilising these non-pharmacological strategies in combination with the pharmacological interventions in order to optimise the multidimensional approach to pain management. Below is a general list of some of the strategies; further complementary strategies for specific conditions will be covered in subsequent chapters.

- **Heat** is frequently used to treat subacute and chronically painful conditions such as musculoskeletal pain prior to exercise and mobilisation. It can be comfort-giving and is usually applied as hot packs, paraffin wax baths or even warm bandages.
- **Cold** in the form of ice packs is used primarily to alter blood flow and the metabolic activity that occurs in acutely injured tissues. This is said to limit oedema and the release of pain-causing chemicals. Cold can also block nerve fibre activity resulting in numbness and thereby limiting the afferent barrage of pain stimulation to the central nervous system. For example, frozen peas wrapped in a damp towel to protect the skin from ice-burn can be very effective after a smack on the nose.
- **Massage** is performed with the mechanical action of hands on skin and subcutaneous structures. It is believed to enhance the circulation of blood and lymph, resulting in an increased supply of oxygen and the removal of waste products and pain-causing chemicals. Massage is also credited with reducing muscular tone and increasing the pain threshold. However, for most people it will reduce the 'unpleasantness' of pain perhaps more by relaxing the mind and reducing anxiety (Ernst 2003; Piotrowski et al. 2003).
- **Comfort strategies** such as positioning pillows and bed linen can make patients feel more relaxed and ease painful limbs. Ensuring that noise and interruptions are minimised in order to provide a relaxing environment conducive to rest is also important. Ambient temperature should be comfortable too.
- Nurses may underestimate the benefits of **presencing** or 'being alongside' and the comfort they bring by staying with a patient who is experiencing pain. Sharing the experience by sitting with the patient whilst waiting for another member of staff to

---

Box 2.3 Skilled companionship

In a seminal book by Morva Fordham and Virginia Dunn entitled *Alongside the Person in Pain* (1994) the authors write passionately about how important and powerful the nurse can be in reducing the experience of pain through 'skilled companionship'. They suggest three key activities for the nurse in this endeavour:

(1) **Entering into the experience and establishing a presence.** The nurse:
  - understands the uniqueness of pain for a person
  - brings an acknowledgement that the pain exists
  - understands how pain is affecting the person
(2) **Sustaining the connection, maintaining the presence**
  - establishing trust
(3) **Helping the person make other connections**
  - communicating with other members of the multidimensional team

---

arrive can give considerable comfort and alleviate the anxiety and sense of isolation that pain brings (Box 2.3).

Physical therapy treatments

These include a range of strategies to help restore function and improve mobility, thereby helping to relieve the pain and stiffness associated with inactivity. There are some suggestions that these therapies may activate endogenous pain pathways but more research is needed.

- **Mobilisation** is usually undertaken by physiotherapists and is designed to improve function by applying oscillating and repetitive movements to joints. It may involve maintaining sustained positions to compress or stretch articular structures (Strong et al. 2002).
- **Manipulation** is usually done at speed without patient control and is associated with joint noise such as a click or crack (Strong et al. 2002).
- **Chiropractic manipulation** usually involves manipulation of the spine, while **osteopathic manipulation** is focused on the whole body system of manual therapy.
- **Exercise** is most often used as a therapy for low back pain. It is said to increase mobility and flexibility whilst restoring confidence and challenging fear avoidance behaviour. Reductions in pain as a result have been reported.

Electrophysical treatments

- **Cryotherapy** is a type of cold therapy to relieve pain, usually in the form of vapocoolant spray or cold packs.
- **Infrared lamps** deliver infrared electromagnetic radiation to heat tissue and are said to improve circulation and reduce pain.
- **Transcutaneous electrical nerve stimulation** (TENS) is still widely used for all types of chronic pain, including neuropathic pain, although its effect beyond placebo is challenged (Bandolier 1997; Carroll et al. 2000). For many patients it offers a drug-free alternative, but more research is needed to give a true picture of its efficacy. Conventional TENS is the most commonly used mode of stimulation. Others include acupuncture-like TENS, brief/intense TENS and burst TENS. The TENS electrodes may be applied directly to the painful area or over the course of the relevant nerve trunks or nerve roots, but never directly on damaged or broken skin. These devices are usually used two to three times a day for no more than about one hour in order to limit the risk of skin irritation. The devices are very safe, but certain contraindications apply. See Fig. 2.7 for examples of typical TENS machines.
- **Spinal stimulation** delivers low voltage electrical stimulation to the spinal cord via implanted electrodes. The stimulation device is intended to block the sensation of pain and is sometimes used for neuropathic pain such as that associated with phantom limb (Cameron 2004).
- **Laser therapy** involves the use of electromagnetic energy to stimulate tissue repair and wound healing. It is used for musculoskeletal, arthrogenic, temporomandibular and neurogenic pain (Turner & Hode 1999; Kulekcioglu et al. 2003).

- **Ultrasound** uses sound rather than electromagnetic energy to stimulate repair following soft tissue injuries involving chronic wounds and ulcers. It is also used for musculoskeletal, arthrogenic and neurogenic pain.

Resources

- Guidelines for the use of spinal stimulation are available from the British Pain Society (www.britishpainsociety.org).
- Regarding low level laser therapy for painful joints see www.jr2.ox.ac.uk/bandolier/band123/b123-5.
- Van Der Windt et al. (2000).

Cognitive behavioural therapy

Cognitive behavioural therapy is now a well recognised and researched strategy for certain conditions, including chronic pain. It combines psychotherapy with behavioural therapy. Behavioural therapy helps to weaken any connections between unpleasant experiences and the patient's habitual reactions to them which may result in self-defeating behaviour. Cognitive therapy teaches patients how certain thinking patterns can cause or emphasise these problems and how to actively alter these.

Cognitive behavioural therapy recognises that the behavioural strategies listed below are important and the therapy involves graded practice and relapse prevention as valid and effective treatment of patients with chronic pain. There is strong evidence to support the effectiveness of these strategies (Morley et al. 1999) which aim to target the following:

- Negative thought patterns such as catastrophising are targeted, with therapists helping patients develop more positive thoughts.
- Negative feelings need to be challenged, as do unhelpful or inaccurate beliefs, in order to assist patients to see their problems as manageable and not overwhelming.
- Maladaptive behaviours such as fear avoidance need to be converted to active involvement with treatment and graded improvements in function.

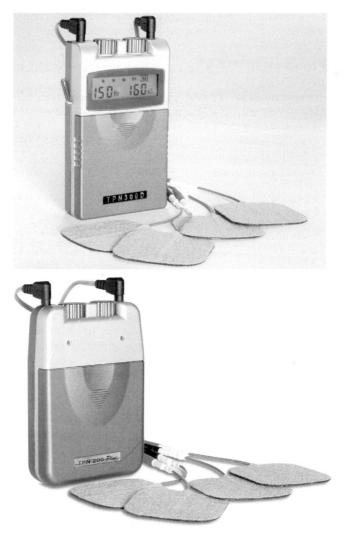

Fig. 2.7 Examples of TENS machines. (Reproduced with kind permission of Physio Med Ltd.)

The following factors are identified as key to the development of cognitive behavioural strategies (Turk & Meichenbaum 1994, p. 1338):

- Individuals are active processors of information and not passive reactors.
- Thoughts such as appraisal, expectations and beliefs can influence mood, affect physiological processes, have social consequences and influence behaviour.
- Behaviour is reciprocal and is determined by the individual as well as his/her environment.
- Individuals can learn to adapt their ways of thinking, feeling and behaving.
- Individuals should be active in changing any maladaptive thoughts, feelings and behaviour.

Other factors that are targeted usually as part of a multidisciplinary cognitive behavioural programme of chronic pain management include:

- Skills development
  — Expectations
  — Self efficacy
  — Coping strategies
- Lifestyle management
  — Goal setting and pacing
  — Relaxation
  — Sleep management
  — Empowerment
  — Social support
  — Family dynamics

Summary

This chapter has explored a range of 'front line' strategies associated with the management of acute and chronic pain. We have emphasised the importance of combining different modalities to exploit the multidimensional nature of pain.

APPENDIX 2.1

Example of an Epidural Observation Chart

Includes the prescription of boluses and top-ups combined with a monitoring and maintenance protocol.

Addressograph	Consultant surgeon: ....
	Ward: ....
	Date: ....
	Anaesthetist: ....

EPIDURAL SOLUTION

Date	Solution	Infusion rate	Signature
	Bupivicaine 0.125% + Fentanyl 4 mcg in sodium chloride 0.9% in 500 ml	2–	
	Bupivicaine 0.1% + Fentanyl 2 mcg in sodium chloride 0.9% in 500 ml	2–	
	Bupivicaine 0.15% in sodium chloride 0.9% in 500 ml	2–	
	3 ml bolus x 3 of epidural solution **authorised staff only** PIRITON 4 mg P.O. or NALOXONE 0.2 mg IM for itching GELOFUSINE 500 ml stat if systolic BP < 80 mmHg		

EXTRA INFUSIONS

Date	Time	Infusion	Signature

BOLUS/TOP-UPS

Date	Time	Solution	Volume	Signature

Observation	Action
Respiratory rate	If respiratory rate is <10/min stop the pump If respiratory rate is <8 stop pump and inform on-call anaesthetist
Blood pressure	If systolic BP is <80 mmHg give gelofusine 500 ml stat
Pain intensity 0 = No pain at rest or on movement 1–4 = No pain at rest or mild pain on movement 5–7 = Moderate pain at rest, severe on moving 8–10 = Severe pain at rest	Pain intensity 1–4 give paracetamol/NSAID if appropriate 5–7 as above and increase epidural infusion 8–10 increase rate and inform APS (on-call anaesthetist out of hours)
Sedation score 0 = Alert patient/normal sleep (rousable) 1 = Mild (occasionally drowsy, rousable) 2 = Moderate (frequently drowsy, easily roused) 3 = Severe (somnolent, difficult to rouse)	If patient is unrousable, stop epidural infusion and inform on-call anaesthetist
Sensation 0 = Normal sensation 1 = Altered sensation (to touch or temperature) 2 = Absence of sensation	If there is any altered sensation of legs (or arms) call APS (on-call anaesthetist out of hours)
Motor power 0 = Normal power 1 = Weakness but can lift against gravity 2 = Cannot move limb against gravity 3 = Cannot move limb	If there is any limb motor weakness call APS (on-call anaesthetist out of hours)
Pruritus (itching) 0 = No pruritus 1 = pruritus 2 = uncomfortable	Administer piriton 4 mg P.O. as first line treatment If no response, consider naloxone 0.2 mg IM

Observations must be recorded:
- Half hourly for 2 hours
- Hourly for 4 hours
- Four hourly thereafter

OBSERVATIONS

Date	Time	Rate ml/hr	Total infused	Pain at rest	Pain on movement	Sedation score	Resp rate	Blood pressure	Sensory Score L R		Motor score L R		Site checked	Comments signature

Date epidural discontinued ....   Signs of infection YES/NO   Tip/swab sent for culture YES/NO

Nurse removing epidural ....

REFERENCES

Averley, P.A., Girdler, N.M., Bond, S., Steen, N. & Steele, J. (2004) A randomised controlled trial of paediatric conscious sedation for dental treatment using conscious sedation combined with inhaled nitrous oxide or nitrous oxide/sevoflurane. *Anaesthesia* **59**, 844–852.

Baird, M.B. & Schug, S.A. (1996) Safety aspect of postoperative pain relief. *Pain Digest* **6** (4), 219–225.

Ballantyne, J.C., Carr, D.B., de Ferranti, S., et al. (1998) The comparative effects of postoperative analgesic therapies on pulmonary outcome: cumulative meta-analysis of randomised controlled trials. *Anaesthesia and Analgesia* **86** (3), 598–612.

Bandolier (1997) *Does TENS Work?* Available at www.jr2.ox.ac.uk/bandolier/band37/b37-3, accessed August 2005.

Bernstein, B.A. & Pachter, L.M. (1993) Cultural considerations in children's pain. In: Schecter, N.K., Berde, C.B. & Yaster, M. (eds) *Pain in Infants, Children and Adolescents*, pp. 113–122. Williams & Wilkins, Baltimore.

Bird, A. & Wallis, M. (2002) Nursing knowledge and assessment skills in the management of patients receiving analgesia via epidural infusion. *Journal of Advanced Nursing* **40** (5), 522–531.

Boezaart, A.P., Eksteen, J.A., Sput, G.V., Rossouw, R. & Knipe, M. (1999) Intrathecal morphine. Double blind evaluation of optimal dosage for analgesia after major lumbar spinal surgery. *Spine* **24** (11), 1131–1137.

Brand, P. & Yancy, P. (1993) *Pain: The Gift Nobody Wants*. Harper Collins, New York. British National Formulary (2004) *British National Formulary*. British Medical Association and Royal Pharmaceutical Society of Great Britain, London.

Bronfort, G., Haas, M., Evans, R.L. & Bouter, L.M. (2004) Efficacy of spinal manipulation and mobilization for low back pain and neck pain: a systematic review and best evidence synthesis. *The Spine Journal* **4** (3), 335–356.

Buskila, D., Neumann, L. & Press, J. (2005) Genetic factors in neuromuscular pain. *CNS Spectrums* **10** (4), 281–284.

Cameron, T. (2004) Safety and efficacy of spinal cord stimulation for the treatment of chronic pain: a 20-year literature review. *Journal of Neurosurgery* **100** (3, Spine), 254–267.

Carroll, D., Moore, R.A., McQuay, H.J., Fairman, F., Tramèr, M. & Leijon, G. (2000) Transcutaneous electrical nerve stimulation (TENS) for chronic pain. *The Cochrane Database of Systematic Reviews* **4**.

Clarke, K.A. & Iphofen, R. (2005) Believing the patient with chronic pain: a review of the literature. *British Journal of Nursing* **14** (9), 490–493.

Davis, N. (1999) Sustained release and enteric coated NSAIDs. *Journal of Pharmacy and Pharmaceutical Science* **2** (1), 5–14.

De Leon-Casasola, O.A. (1996) Clinical outcome after epidural anaesthesia and analgesia in high-risk surgical patients. *Regional Anaesthesia* **21** (Suppl. 6), 144–148.

Ernst, E. (2003) Massage treatment for back pain. *British Medical Journal* **326**, 562–563.

Evans, A. (2003) Use of Entonox in the community for control of procedural pain. *British Journal of Community Nursing* **8** (11), 488–494.

Fordham, M. & Dunn, V. (1994) *Alongside the Person in Pain*. Baillière Tindall, London.

Gilron, I. (2002) Is gabapentin a 'broad-spectrum' analgesic? *Anaesthesiology* **97**, 537–539.

Greenstein, B. (2004) *Clinical Pharmacology for Nurses*, 17th edn. Churchill Livingstone, China.

Jordan, S. & White, J. (2001) Non steroidal anti-inflammatory drugs, clinical issues. *Nursing Standard* **15** (23), 45–54.

Jorgensen, L.N., Rasmussen, L.S., Nielsen, P.T., Leffers, A. & Albrecht-Beste, E. (1991) Antithrombotic efficacy of continuous extradural analgesia after knee replacement. *British Journal of Anaesthesia* **66** (1), 8–12.

Kalso, E.L., Poyhia, R., Onnela, P., Linko, K., Tigerstedt, I. & Tammisto, T. (1991) Intravenous morphine and oxycodone for pain after abdominal surgery. *Acta Anaesthesiologica Scandinavica* **35**, 642.

Keefe, F.J., Affleck, G., France, C.R., et al. (2004) Gender differences in pain, coping, and mood in individuals having osteoarthritic knee pain: a within-day analysis. *Pain* **110** (3), 571–577.

Kehlet, H. (1989) Surgical stress: the role of pain and analgesia. *British Journal of Anaesthesia* **63** (2), 189–195.

Kimble, L.P., McGuire, D.B., Dunbar, S.B., Fazio, S., De, A., Weintraub, W.S. & Strickland, O.S. (2003) Gender differences in pain characteristics of chronic stable angina and perceived physical limitation in patients with coronary artery disease. *Pain* **101** (1–2), 45–53.

Kulekcioglu, S., Sivrioglu, K., Ozcan, O. & Parlak, M. (2003) Effectiveness of low-level laser therapy in temporomandibular disorder. *Scandinavian Journal of Rheumatology* **32** (2), 114–118.

Lui, S.S., Carpenter, R.K., Mackey, D.C., et al. (1995) Effects of perioperative analgesic technique on rate of recovery after colon surgery. *Anaesthesiology* **83** (4), 757–765.

McCaffery, M. & Pasero, C. (1999) *Opioid Analgesics in Pain. Clinical Manual*. Mosby, New York.

Melzack, R. (1999) From the gate to the neuromatrix. *Pain* August (Suppl. 6), S121–S126.

Mitchell, L.A., MacDonald, R.A. & Brodie, E.E. (2004) Temperature and the cold pressor test. *Journal of Pain* **5** (4), 233–237.

Morris, D.B. (1991) *The Culture of Pain*. University of California Press, Berkeley.

Morley, S., Eccleston, C. & Williams, A. (1999) Systematic review of meta-analysis of randomised controlled trials of cognitive behaviour therapy and behaviour therapy for chronic pain in adults, excluding headache. *Pain* **80**, 1–13.

Nederhand, M.J., Hermens, H.J., Ijzerman, M.J., Turk, D.C. & Zilvold, G. (2003) Chronic neck pain disability due to an acute whiplash injury. *Pain* **102** (1–2), 63–71.

Piguet, V., Mesmeules, J. & Dayer, P. (1998) Lack of acetaminophen ceiling effect on R111 nociceptive flexion reflex. *European Journal of Clinical Pharmacology* **53**, 321–324.

Piotrowski, M.M., Paterson, C., Mitchinson, A., Kim, H.M., Kirsh, M. & Hinshaw, D.B. (2003) Massage as adjuvant therapy in the management of acute postoperative pain: a preliminary study in men. *Journal of the American College of Surgeons* **197** (6), 1037–1046.

Rainville, J., Hartigan, C., Martinez, E., Limke, J., Jouve, C. & Finno, M. (2004) Exercise as a treatment for chronic low back pain. *The Spine Journal* **4** (1), 106–115.

Richardson, J. (2001) Post-operative epidural analgesia: introducing evidence-based guidelines through an education and assessment process. *Journal of Clinical Nursing* **10** (2), 238–245.

Sachs, C. (2005) Oral analgesics for acute non-specific pain. *American Family Physician* **71** (5), 913–918.

Scottish Intercollegiate Guidelines Network (SIGN) (2005) *Safe Sedation of Children Undergoing Diagnostic and Therapeutic Procedures. A National Clinical Guideline. Scotland*. Available at www.sign.ac.uk/guidelines, accessed August 2005.

Sealey, L. (2002) Nurse administration of Entonox to manage pain in ward settings. *Nursing Times* **98** (46), 28–29.

Strong, J., Unruh, A.M., Wright, A. & Baxter, G.D. (eds) (2002) *Pain: A Textbook for Therapists*. Churchill Livingstone, London.

Thomas, K.S., Muir, K.R., Doherty, M., Jones, A.C., O'Reilly, S.E. & Bassey, E.J. (2002) Home based exercise programme for knee pain and knee osteoarthritis: randomised controlled trial. *British Medical Journal* **325**, 752.

Turk, D.C. & Meichenbaum, D. (1994) A cognitive-behavioural approach to pain management. In: Wall P.D. & Melzack, R. (eds) *Textbook of Pain*, 3rd edn, pp. 1337–1418. Churchill Livingstone, Edinburgh.

Turner, J. & Hode, L. (1999) *Low Level Laser Therapy. Clinical Practice and Scientific Background*. Prima Books, Grangeberg, Sweden.

Unruh, A.M. (1996) Gender variations in clinical pain. *Pain* **65**, 123–167.

Unruh, A.M. (1997) Why can't a woman be more like a man? *Behavioural and Brain Sciences* **20**, 467–468.

Unruh, A.M. & Campbell, M.A. (1999) Gender variation in children's pain experience. In: McGrath, P.J. & Finley, G.A. (eds) Chronic and recurrent pain in children and adolescents. *Progress in Pain Research and Management* **13**, 199–241.

Unruh, A.M. & McGrath, P.J. (2000) Pain in children: psychosocial issues. In: Melville, J. & Wright, V. (eds) Pediatric rheumatological diseases. *Rheumatological Rehabilitation Series* **3**, 141–168.

Unruh, A.M., Ritchie, J.A. & Merskey, H. (1999) Does gender affect appraisal of pain and pain coping strategies? *Clinical Journal of Pain* **15**, 31–40.

Vaile, J.H. & Davis, P. (1998) Topical NSAIDs for musculoskeletal conditions. *Drugs* **56**, 783–799.

Van Der Windt, D.A., Van Der Heijden, G.J., Van Den Berg, S.G., Ter Riet, G., De Winter, A.F. & Bouter, L.M. (2000) Ultrasound therapy for acute ankle sprains. *Cochrane Database Systematic Reviews*. Available at www.mrw.interscience.wiley.com/cochrane/clsysrev/articles/cd001250/frame.

Vickers, M.D., O'Flaherty, D., Szekely, S.M., Read, M. & Yshizumi, J. (1992) Tramadol: pain relief by an opioid without depression of respiration. *Anaesthesia* **47**, 291–296.

Zborowski, M. (1952) Cultural components in responses to pain. *Journal of Social Issues* **8**, 16–30.

Pain in Neonates and Infants (0–6 months)

3

INTRODUCTION

This chapter discusses the complexity of managing pain in preterm neonates to 6 month old babies. As recently as the late 1970s and early 1980s analgesia for infants was given little importance as it was assumed that their nervous systems were too immature for them to experience pain. Papers were published on anaesthetic techniques for cardiac surgery where no analgesia at all was administered. We now accept that this treatment was inhumane. Research has indicated that the neuropeptides, monoamines and catecholamines implicated in the pain pathways are present at birth (Loughnan & Ahluwalia 1997). Neonates also have the neuronal apparatus to detect painful stimuli, but perhaps in a less organised way than adults (Fitzgerald 1993). That they can exhibit both behavioural and physiological responses to painful procedures is now no longer in doubt (McCulloch et al. 1995).

However, despite our increasing understanding of the development of pain pathways, neonates, especially those who are preterm neonates, remain under-medicated for pain, even when undergoing frequent painful procedures (Johnston et al. 1997). Misconceptions continue regarding the inability of neonates to experience pain and the safety of analgesics or anaesthetics administered during the neonatal period (Anand 2001). Contemporary research findings suggest that pain relief is an imperative, besides ethical and humane obligation; there may be long-term and potentially permanent consequences from painful sensory stimulation on the development of pain pathways in the nervous system (Sternberg et al. 2005). These discoveries suggest that pain management for tiny babies should strive to be even more effective.

LEARNING OBJECTIVES

❏ To discuss some of the challenges to effective pain management for neonates and infants
❏ To identify some of the common causes of infant pain
❏ To recognise the additional factors that complicate pain assessment in neonates and infants
❏ To explore several interventions that may be appropriate to reduce pain

ACUTE PAIN

Principles of assessment and evaluation for acute pain

The importance of assessing neonatal and infant pain cannot be stressed enough. Neonates cannot verbalise their pain and rely on others to recognise, assess and manage their pain. Health care professionals can diagnose neonatal pain only by recognising the neonate's behavioural and physiological response to noxious stimuli. Often parental involvement in this can prove invaluable to help interpret responses to pain.

For infant pain assessment to be effective it needs to be regular and repeated using a tool that staff are able to interpret as clearly as possible. None of the existing tools fulfils all criteria for an ideal measure and different pain assessment tools may work in different circumstances for different reasons (Duhn & Medves 2004). It may also be necessary to individualise an existing tool depending on clinical circumstances. Many of the assessment tools have been developed for research studies to evaluate interventions. The requirements for using this type of tool may be very different to those of the busy neonatal nurse in the clinical setting. Below are listed just some of the behavioural and physiological indicators of pain that can be used.

Behavioural indicators of pain
• Facial expression
• Body movements
• Crying

Physiological indicators of pain
• Heart rate
• Respiratory rate

- Blood pressure
- Oxygen saturation (SaO$_2$)
- Vagal tone
- Palmar sweating
- Plasma cortisol or catecholamine levels

It is important to ensure that all staff are using exactly the same criteria to measure pain and distress and for this reason we recommend the use of a formal assessment tool. There are several validated and reliable pain measures available to assess acute pain in term and preterm neonates. Below are some examples, including CRIES and NIPS mentioned by the American Association of Paediatrics, and TPPPS (Tarbell et al. 1992), DEGR (Gauvain-Piquard et al. 1987) and CHEOPS (McGrath et al. 1985) mentioned in the Royal College of Nursing guidelines (RCN 2005).

Examples of pain assessment tools

For comprehensive reviews of these neonatal assessment tools see Duhn & Medves (2004) and the Royal College of Nursing's website: www.rcn.org.uk/publications/pdf/guidelines/cpg_contents.pdf.

- **Pain Rating Scale (PRS) 1994 Infants**: 1–12 months of age (Joyce et al. 1994)
- **Riley Infant Pain Scale (RIPS) 1996**: postoperative infants and children (Schade et al. 1996)
- **Maximally Discriminative Facial Movement Coding System (MAX) 1995**: infants 0–2 years (Izard 1995)
- **Infant Body Coding System (IBCS) 1993**: preterm and full-term newborns (Craig et al. 1993)
- **Neonatal Pain and Discomfort Scale (EDIN) 2001**: preterm infants, average gestational age 31.5 weeks (Debillon et al. 2001)
- **Clinical Scoring System (CSS) 1987 or (POPS) 1996**: infants from 1 to 7 months requiring surgery (Schade et al. 1996)
- **Modified Postoperative Comfort Score (PCS) 1998 revision of POPS**: mechanically ventilated preterm infants (Guinsburg et al. 1998)
- **Behavioural Pain Score 1994**: mechanically ventilated preterm infants (Pokela et al. 1994)

- **Modified Behavioural Pain Scale (MBPS) 1995**: healthy infants 4–6 months (Taddio et al. 1995)
- **Baby Facial Action Coding System (Baby FACS) 1988**: healthy newborns (Rosenstein & Oster 1988)
- **Children's and Infants' Postoperative Pain Scale (CHIPPS) 2000**: newborns, infants and young children (Buttner & Finke 2002)
- **Acute Pain Rating Scale for Neonates 1997**: newborns between 25 and 41 weeks gestational age (Carbajal et al. 1997)
- **Liverpool Infant Distress Scale (LIDS) 1996**: newborn infants postoperatively (see Appendix 1 at the end of this chapter) (Horgan & Choonara 1996)
- **Neonatal Facial Coding System (NFCS) 1998**: preterm infants and well newborns (Grunau et al. 1998; Peters et al. 2003)
- **Bernese Pain Scale for Neonates (BPSN) 2004)**: term and preterm neonates with and without CPAP ventilation (Cignacco et al. 2004)
- **The Pain Assessment Tool (PATS) 1994**: neonates; and **2005**: critically ill ventilated infants in a neonatal intensive care unit (Hodgkinson et al. 1994; Spence et al. 2005)
- **The Neonatal Pain Assessment Tool 1995**: infants in an intensive care setting (Friedrichs et al. 1995)
- **The Scale for Use in Newborns (SUN) 1998**: preterm and term infants during procedures (Blauer & Gertsmann 1998)
- **The Distress Scale for Ventilated Newborn Infants (DSVNI) 1996**: initial reporting of tool development (Sparshott 1996)
- **The Comfort Scale 1992 and 2005**: newborns to young children (Ambuel et al. 1992; van Dijk et al. 2005)
- **The CRIES 1995**: infants postoperatively (Krechel & Bildner 1995)
- **The Neonatal Infant Pain Scale (NIPS) 1993, 2002 and 2003**: preterm and term infants (Lawrence et al. 1993; Hudson-Barr et al. 2002; Gallo 2003)
- **The Pain Assessment in Neonates (PAIN) Scale 2002**: neonates with gestational ages 26–47 weeks (Hudson-Barr et al. 2002)
- **The Modified Infant Pain Scale (MIPS) 1998**: healthy term infants undergoing elective surgery (Buchholz et al. 1998)
- **The Premature Infant Pain Profile (PIPP) 1996**: infants from 28 to 40 gestation (Stevens et al. 1996)

- **The Children's Hospital of Eastern Ontario Pain Scale (CHEOPS) 1985**: neonates (McGrath et al. 1985)

Physiological changes
In their first 6 months many babies will experience bouts of colic and the discomfort of teething, conditions that most parents learn to manage early on if a good sleep pattern is to be established. However, some neonates will experience significant pain associated with prematurity, congenital abnormalities or ill health. These painful stimuli may not always come from major surgery to correct a serious congenital malformation but from more trivial sources such as repeated heal pricks to collect blood samples. The management of this 'inflicted' or 'procedural' pain is covered later in this chapter.

Colic
Colic is often the term given for babies who cry for longer than 3 hours every day. The causes of colic are not known and extended crying in a baby who is otherwise healthy and well fed, although distressing for parents, may not indicate any significant organic problem. About 20% of babies get colic, usually beginning at around 2–4 weeks of age and lasting for 3 months or longer. In the past it was thought to be related to the digestive system and trapped wind, although there is little evidence to indicate that gastrointestinal problems are the principal source of this pain. An immature nervous system rather than actual nociceptive pain is sometimes suggested as a cause with a baby unable to regulate crying once it starts.

Pharmacological strategies
Drugs are not usually recommended for this condition, although preparations such as 'gripe water' available without a prescription may help to relieve some symptoms. Dimeticone (e.g. Infacol) is also available to help relieve trapped wind if this is suspected.

Non-pharmacological strategies
These suggestions are first-line strategies and parents will usually find one or two that prove helpful:

Box 3.1 Research into the treatment of colic

A systematic review was undertaken to evaluate the effectiveness of diets, drug treatment and behavioural interventions of infants who experience colic. Following database searches 27 controlled trials were identified. The advice to reduce stimulation was beneficial, whereas the advice to increase carrying and holding seemed not to reduce crying. Elimination of cows' milk protein was effective when substituted by hypoallergenic formula milks, but effectiveness of substitution by soy formula milks was unclear when only trials of sound methodological quality were considered. The researchers concluded that infants with colic should preferably be treated by advising carers to reduce stimulation and with a one-week trial of a hypoallergenic formula milk (Lucassen et al. 1998).

- Trying a different formula for bottle-fed babies.
- For breast-fed babies, omitting certain foods in the maternal diet such as cabbage, broccoli, cauliflower, sprouts, parsnips, beans, onions, garlic, apricots, melon, spicy foods, caffeine and alcohol.
- If there is a family history of milk sugar (lactose) intolerance, breastfeeding mothers may try eliminating cows' milk and dairy produce from their diet.
- If the baby seems to have a lot of wind, make sure he or she is burped frequently. For bottle-fed babies try a change of feeding position or a bottle and teat designed to reduce the amount of air the baby swallows during a feed.
- Carry the baby securely wrapped in a sling or back pack.
- Leave the baby near a continuous noise or vibration such as a dishwasher.
- A car journey or push chair ride.
- A dummy or pacifier.
- Gentle stomach or back massage.
- A warm water bath.
- Try to reduce parental anxiety!

Box 3.1 provides information on some research into infant colic.

Resources

- A BUPA fact sheet for parents and carers: www.hcd2.bupa.co.uk, search under Infant colic
- The National Childbirth Trust: www.nctpregnancyandbabycare.com
- Helpline for families having difficulty with a crying baby: Tel. 020 74045011

Surgery

The following are some examples of the more common surgical procedures undertaken on neonates and infants:

- Infant circumcision
- First stage hypospadias (abnormal opening of urethra) repair
- Laparotomy for repair of exomphalus (projection of abdominal organs through the umbilicus), intersusscception (an obstruction caused by part of the intestine sliding into the section of intestine immediately beneath it like a closing telescope), volvulus (an obstruction caused by a loop of bowel twisting around itself), pyloric stenosis (a narrowing of the muscular exit from the stomach to the duodenum), Hirschsprung's disease (resulting in extreme dilatation of the colon), incarcerated hernia
- Repair of congenital heart defects, e.g. patent ductus arteriosus
- Repair of tracheo-oesophageal fistula
- Repair of diaphragmatic hernia
- Ventriculoperitoneal shunt, used to relieve fluid pressure buildup in the brain. It involves implanting a draining tube from the ventricles in the brain to channel the excess cerebrospinal fluid into the peritoneum
- First stage cleft palate surgery

Experiencing short stay postoperative pain – circumcision

Case study

Rupert aged 5 days is admitted to hospital to undergo a routine neonatal circumcision as a matter of parental choice. He is fit and healthy following a normal delivery at term at home. He is the first child of Paul and Anita and they have been anxious about their decision. He has been breastfed and seems a happy and contented baby. Anita will stay with him for the duration of his stay.

Although this procedure may now be less common in the UK, in the USA it remains the most frequently performed surgical procedure during the newborn period. This is despite the 1999

American Academy of Paediatrics (AAP 1999) policy statement indicating that it is unnecessary. What is perhaps more alarming is that it is still performed in some instances with no anaesthesia, instead citing 'concern over adverse drug effects' and 'the procedure does not warrant anaesthesia' (Stang & Snellman 1998).

Pharmacological strategies

Local anaesthesia
Local anaesthesia given as a regional block or infiltration has been shown to provide the most effective form of pain control. The most common procedures undertaken are dorsal penile nerve and circumferential ring blocks using local anaesthetics such as 1 or 2% lignocaine or 0.25% or 0.5% bupivacaine without adrenalin (Williamson 1997; Hardwick-Smith et al. 1998; Stang et al. 1988). The pain relief that local anaesthetics can offer has been shown to relieve both the stress and the pain of circumcision, which manifests as:

- Smaller decreases in transcutaneous oxygen saturation level
- Decreased crying time
- Smaller increases in heart rate
- Lower elevations in serum cortisol level (Kraft 2003)

Minimising pain associated with infiltration of lignocaine has not been evaluated in infants, but in adults buffering the solution with sodium bicarbonate, warming it, injecting slowly and using a very small needle may reduce the distress this can cause (Armel & Horowitz. 1994; Lugo-Janer et al. 1994; Stang et al. 1997).

Topical local anaesthetics
Several studies have evaluated the use of topical anaesthetic creams for circumcision, with the majority of studies being conducted using a lidocaine-prilocaine cream EMLA (eutectic mixture of local anaesthetics). This has been shown to be effective (Taddio et al. 1997a, 1997b, 2000; Mohan et al. 1998; Joyce et al. 2001), but a topical preparation does not appear to be as effective as a penile nerve block. A local anaesthetic cream, however, may also be used to decrease the pain during needle insertion when infants are going on to have a block. A practical disadvan-

tage of EMLA is that it must be applied to the skin of the penis with an occlusive dressing for 60–90 minutes before a procedure. EMLA is not recommended as the sole method of pain control for neonatal circumcision but may be useful as part of a multimodal approach. EMLA should be used cautiously in the neonate owing to reports of methaemoglobinaemia (reduced oxygen-carrying capacity) associated with its use (Frayling et al. 1990).

Paracetamol
Paracetamol is the mainstay of postoperative pain management, but given 1–2 hours preoperatively in the usual dose of 10–15 mg/kg by mouth it has not been shown to be effective for circumcision (Howard et al. 1994; Macke 2001). Again there is also a slight theoretical risk of methaemoglobinaemia with concurrent use of paracetamol and EMLA (Zenk et al. 2000).

Non-pharmacological strategies
Many studies have tried to evaluate the effectiveness of non-pharmacological interventions for circumcision and found them to be ineffective when used alone. Thus it is important to integrate them with other pharmacological approaches and thereby offer a balanced analgesic approach. In the first instance, parental information and reassurance are vital (Box 3.2).

Sucrose
The use of oral sucrose has been quite extensively studied and shown to reduce the behavioural responses to circumcision pain.

Box 3.2 Parental concern and distress over infant pain

196 parents with infants who were admitted to neonatal units completed questionnaires concerning infant pain, parental stress and anxiety. Parents reported that their infants experienced moderate to severe pain and this was greater than they had expected ($p < 0.001$). Only 4% of parents received written information, while 58% reported that they received verbal information about infant pain. Only 18% of parents reported that they were shown signs of infant pain, but 55% were shown how to comfort their infant. Parents had numerous worries about pain and pain treatments. **Conclusions:** parents have unmet information needs about infant pain and wanted greater involvement in their infant's pain care. Parent concerns about infant pain may contribute to parental stress.

See Frank et al. (2004) for further information.

It is thought to produce analgesia via both endogenous opioid and non-opioid pathways (Stevens et al. 2001) as its effects can be reversed with naloxone. It is usually given as a 24–25% concentration in water.

Dummies
Dummies or pacifiers are generally used to calm a crying baby and when used with sucrose appear to provide additional pain relief during circumcision (Gunnar et al. 1984; Herschel et al. 1998)

Positioning
Lying an infant in a flat, unflexed position on an operating table also appears to cause additional distress during circumcision. The use of a special padded chair-like device has shown a 50% reduction in distress, indicating that comfort and security is also a feature of infant pain control (Stang et al. 1997). Swaddling the infant with light blankets can provide comfort.

Sound
The results of using various sounds such as classical music and intra-uterine noises played to infants during circumcision pain have been mixed, although one small study did indicate some benefit (Joyce et al. 2001).

Feeding
Infants are routinely fasted before circumcision to reduce the risk of vomiting. Ironically infants may vomit as a response to pain during an unanaesthetised circumcision (Lander et al. 1997). As hunger in infants can add to distress and discomfort it is now reported that it may well be safe to discontinue routine fasting (Stang 1997). Neurologically intact infants have numerous reflexive mechanisms to protect their airway during vomiting and aspiration is rare (Jeffery et al. 2000).

Speed, technique and equipment
A number of different instruments can be used to perform circumcision, but a quick procedure by a competent practitioner appears to reduce pain and stress (Taeusch et al. 2002).

Resources

- Razmus et al. (2004) for further information on circumcision pain
- Tibboel et al. (2005) for further information on pharmacological treatments. Weise & Nahata (2005) review several double-blind randomised, placebo-controlled studies using EMLA cream for various procedures performed on infants
- There is some excellent material on pain management during circumcision available via Medscape which offers free registration by following links from their home page www.medscape.com/home

Experiencing long stay postoperative pain – thoracotomy

Case study

Ann is aged 6 weeks and undergoing a thoracotomy for repair of a congenital heart defect (CHD). She is relatively strong and was delivered by caesarean section at term. Her parents are very attentive and extremely anxious. They are particularly concerned about managing any analgesia and medications once Ann is discharged home.

The incidence of congenital heart defect (CHD) is 0.8%, and 25% of these infants will require an intervention soon after birth (Clark 1995; McElhinney & Wernovsky 2001). Parents are vital partners in managing postoperative pain in very young babies, although they may not always recognise their role. Most parents will experience a mixture of shock, disbelief, fear, anger and sadness on discovering they have a baby with a congenital heart defect. However, being able to recognise and report when they think their baby is in pain will help parents feel they are taking an active part in their baby's recovery.

In the past parents assumed that all that could be done was being done (Unruh 2002), but if parents do not challenge the quality of their baby's care and pain control, then there is no incentive for improvement (McGrath & Unruh 1993). How their baby's pain is managed in the perioperative period may be vital to his or her long-term outlook. A good pain assessment tool will help to ensure that treatable pain is not ignored and visiting parents may have the time and motivation to contribute to pain assessment, thus helping to ensure it is carried out regularly.

Pharmacological strategies

Analgesia in the neonate and infant less than 6 months old will always be complicated by the following problems:

- Clinical trials of analgesics are more difficult to conduct in infants due to ethical concerns related to consent, cost of the trial and the relatively small 'market' for analgesics.
- Many pharmacological preparations for adults are not licensed and are untested for neonates and infants.
- Pharmaceutical companies indicate different age limits for their drugs that may not be scientifically justified but may lead to children receiving a subtherapeutic dose of analgesia.
- Pharmacokinetics in infants may be quite different to adults on whom drugs are tested.

Strong opioids

In the ventilated infant or in an environment where close monitoring can take place opioid analgesics such as morphine, fentanyl, diamorphine and sufentanyl are available and effective to treat severe pain (Loughnan & Ahluwalia 1997). These drugs are very effective and must be at the front line of peri- and postoperative pain management following major surgery.

Perioperative opioid management is most commonly achieved with a fentanyl or morphine loading dose intraoperatively and postoperatively via a nurse operated patient controlled analgesia (NPCA) or nurse controlled analgesia (NCA) with a background infusion, or an opioid infusion or included in an epidural infusion selected according to age and development (Gaukroger 1997).

Pre-emptive morphine infusions, additional morphine and lower gestational age are associated with hypotension in preterm neonates. Morphine can still be used safely for most preterm neonates but should be used very cautiously for 23–26 week neonates and those with pre-existing hypotension (Nandi & Fitzgerald 2005).

Midazolam

Midazolam is sometimes used with an opioid for its opioid sparing effects for infants who require sedation and analgesia, but there is little written about this combination. Research with oral midazolam shows that the ability to metabolise and excrete is markedly decreased in preterm infants compared with older children (de Wildt et al. 2002).

Paracetamol

Paracetamol for infants has also not been well studied and it is only recommended in the British National Formulary (BNF 2005) for babies over 2 months for postimmunisation pyrexia. Theoretically neonates may be less susceptible to hepatotoxicity because they produce lower levels of potentially toxic metabolites (Anand et al. 1993). The pharmacokinetics and pharmacodynamics of paracetamol differ substantially in neonates and infants from that in older children and adults; hence, dosing should be adjusted accordingly. There is little research on the pharmacokinetics of paracetamol in premature infants; therefore the general principle of giving lower doses or a longer dosage interval should apply (Loughnan & Ahluwalia 1997).

NSAIDs

Traditional indomethacin tended to be used postoperatively following repair of a patent ductus arteriosus (PDA), but concerns about hepatotoxicity have led to suggestions that ibuprofen may be the safer option without compromising pain control (Pen-Hua et al. 2003; Fanos et al. 2005). Ibuprofen is approved for children of 6 months or over (7 kg) in the British National Formulary (2005) but not for neonates. The use of ibuprofen has been studied in neonates and appears to be safe (Lesko & Mitchell 1995, 1999), although extreme caution is advocated in infants less than 2 months for fear of masking or delaying the investigation of neonatal sepsis. Aspirin is no longer recommended for infants or children because of the risk of Reye's syndrome.

Local anaesthetic drugs

These drugs may well be particularly useful for neonates as they can be safer, produce profound analgesia with a lack of sedation and can provide a long duration of action. Most commonly used are bupivacaine and lignocaine. Where local vasoconstriction is not contraindicated adrenalin may be added to increase safety.

However, even low doses of these drugs if given intravascularly may cause convulsions and cardiac arrest.

Epidural and spinal analgesia

Thoracotomy may result in intense postoperative pain, which may compromise respiratory function and interfere with recovery. Spinal and epidural analgesia have been studied in neonates in an attempt to illustrate the benefits and also to find the ideal drug combinations (Wolf et al. 1998). Continuous epidural analgesia using the caudal approach for patent ductus arteriosus repair has also been advocated (Lin et al. 1999).

Nurse operated patient controlled analgesia (NPCA) pump

Morphine is the most commonly used opioid in PCAs as it has the most pharmacokinetic data available regarding its use. Fentanyl is sometimes used and both these drugs would be prescribed according to the infant's weight. Most hospitals find that it is more convenient to vary the amount of opioid added to the syringe, with the volume of the bolus doses remaining constant rather than reducing the volume of the bolus dose. This is due to the fact that most PCA machines need at least a 0.5 ml volume to be accurate. NPCAs with possibly a background infusion tend to be used in older infants and children as in the newborn great care has to be taken with any bolus dose. Even a loading dose should be given over a period of time, often 30 minutes, as rapid intravenous infusion may lead to acute respiratory depression and hypotension. A continuous infusion is usually the method of choice for tiny infants.

Infusions

The half-life of morphine can vary widely in neonates, from 6 to 8 hours during the first week of life, longer if the neonate is ill and even longer – about 10 hours – in preterm infants (Loughnan & Ahluwalia 1997). Doses need to be selected and monitored with great care, but adequate analgesia appears to be achievable with an infusion rate of 20 µg/kg per hour in ventilated patients and 10–15 µg/kg in spontaneously breathing infants (Levene & Quinn 1992).

Resources

- Ansermino et al. (2003) is useful for a systematic review of non-opioid additives to local anaesthetic for caudal block
- Hansen et al. (1999) and Arana et al. (2001) for paracetamol in infants
- Koroglu et al. (2005) for information on spinal anaesthesia
- Sabrine & Sinha (2000) for general information on pain in the neonate

Non-pharmacological strategies

Non-pharmacological strategies associated with little risk combined with pharmacological methods of pain relief are not always used, even where analgesia in infants may be challenging. McGrath & Unruh (1993) suggest that denial and desensitisation of health care professionals are possible reasons for this. Denial that neonates experience pain and desensitisation of nurses in particular may occur because nurses cannot socially connect with a sick neonate. Pain assessment relies on communication and the sick neonate does not reciprocate in this interaction and so may be offered less attention. Nurses may feel powerless to intervene if they are given only a very limited choice of strategies. The picture is even bleaker for neurologically impaired infants, who appear to receive even less analgesia than non-damaged infants (Stevens et al. 2003).

In addition to sucrose and dummies, the following may be beneficial, particularly during the procedures that babies in the postoperative period may have to undergo as part of routine monitoring.

Breastfeeding

Breastfeeding whilst babies undergo venepuncture and heel stick has been suggested as an effective intervention (Carbajal et al. 2003). Breast milk delivered via syringe is not an effective analgesic so it may be skin-to-skin contact or the sucking itself that offers an analgesic effect (Bucher et al. 2000).

Rocking, holding and cuddling

These measures have been studied and shown to be beneficial for repeated postoperative procedures such as heel prick (Gormally et al. 2003).

Inflicted pain

> **Case study**
>
> Colin was born 7 weeks prematurely and is now aged 2 months. He has remained in hospital since birth and is currently in the neonatal intensive care unit. Because he remains in poor health he has had to undergo repeated traumatic invasive procedures such as venepuncture, lumbar puncture and catheterisation.

Many neonates who are ill receive numerous episodes of 'procedural' pain in the course of their care. Sometimes just the act of turning a neonate or changing his or her nappy can be painful. Examples of the sort of painful procedures carried out on hospitalised neonates and infants are as follows:

- Intravenous cannulation
- Venepuncture
- Peripheral arterial line insertion
- Central venous line insertion
- Chest drain insertion
- Lumbar puncture
- Urethral catheterisation

Ensuring the neonate has periods of rest and is undisturbed can be beneficial. It is also important to critically review the need for investigations in order to avoid unnecessary distress.

Pharmacological strategies
There is little in the way of literature specifically on procedural or inflicted pain in infants and neonates although there is more in older children. The general principles that applied to circumcision may be helpful in highlighting the benefits of using local anaesthetic gels and creams.

EMLA cream
Each 1 g of EMLA contains 25 mg of lignocaine and 25 mg of prilocaine mixed with polyoxyethylene hydrogenated castor oil, carboxypolymethylene, sodium hydroxide and purified water. This

formulation enables a high concentration of local anaesthetic to penetrate superficial tissues. It is usually applied 1 hour prior to a potentially painful procedure such as venepuncture and the cream is covered with an occlusive dressing. The potential side effect of prilocaine, a component of EMLA cream, is methaemaglobinaemia in infants of less than 3 months of age (Phillips 1995). It is therefore suggested that Ametop gel may be more appropriate for neonates, especially preterm (Woolfson et al. 1990).

Ametop gel
This is a semitransparent gel containing 4% w/w amethocaine, purified water, sodium chloride, potassium phosphate, xanthan gum (E415), sodium hydroxide, sodium methyl and propyl-p-hydroxybenzoates (E217 and E219). Each tube contains 1.5 g of gel providing 40 mg amethocaine. The gel is usually left in situ for 30–45 minutes covered with an occlusive dressing and the effect can last for 4–6 hours.

Non-pharmacological strategies
Breastfeeding, rocking and cuddling may not be possible during the more invasive procedures such as venepuncture. However, the following may be employed in addition to appropriate medication:

- Talk in a quiet and calm voice
- Hold the baby securely and comfortably close to your body if possible
- Use dummies and consider adding sucrose
- Distract with music, mobiles, bright coloured toys, etc.
- Involve the parents and carers, if they wish, wherever possible.

Resources

- Gradin et al. (2002) for information on oral glucose
- Moore (2001) for information on amethocaine
- Weise & Nahata (2005) for information on EMLA cream
- Mathew & Mathew (2003) for information on assessment and management of pain in infants

CHRONIC PAIN

There is very little literature available at present on chronic pain in infants although theoretically they may be at risk of chronic pain associated with chronic ill health or a congenital malformation such as hip dysplasia. Neurological defects might also give rise to long-term pain. In the absence of specialist research and literature, the advice would be to carefully monitor for potential pain, treat as for acute pain and evaluate regularly.

SUMMARY

We now know that untreated pain has prolonged physiological and behavioural consequences for newborns. As a group they probably pose the greatest challenge to those health care professionals given the task of controlling their pain, but the rewards can be great not only for the infant but also for parents and staff. The short-term benefits of using opioids on the newborn on ventilators have been demonstrated with improved haemodynamic stability. There is no doubt at all that as the mechanisms underlying the experience of pain become better understood, particularly in the neonate and infant, so too will the need to ensure that pain is recognised and treated appropriately. Professional ignorance should not burden the infant with the potential damage of untreated pain in later life. Recognising situations that elicit pain and distress, accurately assessing the pain and utilising pharmacological and non-pharmacological interventions should become a routine part of care for neonates and infants.

APPENDIX 3.1
LIVERPOOL INFANT DISTRESS SCORE

Reproduced with kind permission of Dr M.F. Horgan, John Moores University, Liverpool, with acknowledgements to Professor S. Glenn (John Moores University Liverpool) and Professor I. Choonara (Derbyshire Children's Hospital, Derby).

Spontaneous motor activity with sucking

Score
0. Completely still but relaxed. Slow movements of head from side to side. Arms and legs stretching and recurling. Elbows

and knees, frog-like, arms away from body. Yawning or smacking lips. Sucking will be energetic and sustained, retaining dummy in mouth. May have spontaneous 'startles' during which baby does not wake.

1. Wriggling and squirming main trunk. Arms and legs extending and recurling at a ratio of 50:50 with (0) type movements. Sucking is energetic, baby chewing on dummy, stops, may cry, then chew again. Dummy usually remains in mouth during crying but if it falls out and is replaced it is accepted immediately.

2. Restless agitation. Spates of quick, sharp movements. Legs move up and down (may be one at a time). Crawling if on tummy. Arms move in front of body, then settle and are still. Ratio of 75:25 with (1) in 10-minute assessment. If sucking, this will not be sustained. Dummy falls out frequently – cry to suck 75:25% of time. If dummy is replaced, baby takes a while to fix.

3. Sharp, tense movements. Quick thrashing of arms and legs, legs more than arms. Fists held clenched, head slightly back. Will only take dummy after much persuasion and then does not sustain sucking. Too much crying to co-ordinate properly.

4. Sharp, tense movements of rigidly held body. Guarding of certain body areas with arms and knees. Fists clenched tightly. Chin shrunk down on to chest. A closing in of the baby on itself, as though to protect. Amount of movement diminishing with very little attempt to retain dummy or to suck.

5. Almost completely still and tense. Holding body guardedly. Thumb inside tightly clenched fist. Does not take dummy at all, conserving energy to breathe, which will be distress-type gasps. No blinking and little eye movement.

Spontaneous excitability

Score

0. Slow, gentle reactions/movements, no cry or jitteriness, may be unmoving.

1. Blinks and slightly screws up face transiently. Mild movements for 10 seconds at a time, then resettles – may not really wake if asleep.

2. Either 1 to 5 episodes of mild jittery type movements without crying, or one startle-type reflex without crying in 10-minute assessment. Settles quite quickly and is at rest in between.
3. Between 5 and 10 episodes of jittery type movements without crying, or one startle-type reflex with a cry in 10-minute assessment. Settles quite quickly and is at rest in between.
4. All reactions/movements are excitable/hyperactive. Almost continuous movements associated with crying. Arms held up and away from body, shaking.
5. Very jumpy and jittery continually. Arms and legs extended during movements and held tensely. Weak cries with movements.

Flexion of fingers and toes

Score
0. Fingers loosely curled as round a pencil. Thumb outside fist. Toes straight and together.
1. Intermittent relaxing and curling of digits.
2. Digits partly curled in more acutely than '0' score and held that way for some minutes.
3. Fingers **OR** toes held tightly curled.
4. Fingers spread out rigid and extended. Feet pointed downwards and held stiffly. Toes curled down tightly.
5. Tightly clenched fist continuously – thumb inside fist. Toes curled downwards, feet turned upwards at sharp angle to leg. **Space between big toe and other toes.**

Tone

Score
0. Relaxed. Arms and legs open and away from body, either spread out or frog-like, if baby on tummy. Elbows and knees at about 45° to arms and legs.
1. Intermittent relaxing and tightening of limbs.
2. Arms and legs held stiffly. Fists clenched or fingers fully extended and stiff. Elbows bent tightly. If on tummy, knees drawn up and arms as (1) but continuously, without relaxation.
3. Limbs held rigidly, knees drawn up, fluctuating with whole body being held rigidly and knees straight.

4. Whole body held taut. Knees held straight. Arms held stiffly close to body, continuously. If the baby moves, whole stance remains taut.

Cry quantity

Score
In each 10-minute assessment:

0. No cry.
1. Small, short bursts of grumbling up to three times in 10 minutes, about 1 minute total crying.
2. 2–4 minutes spent crying either in bursts or as a fairly continuous lusty cry, one-fifth total time of assessment.
3. 4–6 minutes spent crying, two-fifths total time of assessment.
4. 6–8 minutes almost continual cry, two-thirds total time of assessment.
5. 8–10 minutes continuous, almost all time.

Cry quality

Score
0. Neutral vocalisation – occasional short mutter, low pitch. May be absent altogether.
1. Grumbling low pitch about 10 second duration. Stops/starts. Mouth closed – a 'beginning to cry' cry forced from the chest. May settle and stop or proceed.
2. A cross, moderately pitched, lusty cry. Imperative tone to it – intended to signal. Builds up to a crescendo. May stop and start, pauses anticipating a response.
3. A higher pitched wail, quicker to reach crescendo, more sustained and uncomfortable. A siren-like cry, insistent and without pauses.
4. Shocked, startled sudden start to cry. An intense, abrasive hard, high-pitched, piercing cry. Long and sustained then may settle and start again without external provocation (e.g. noise). Tense 'cupping' to tongue. May have breath holding on inspiration.
5. Mewing, pitiable cry. Few and interspersed – may alternate with (4). A chopping quality may be present due to the baby's hyperventilated breathing rate.

Sleep

Score

In a one-hour period majority of type determines score.

0. Greater than 10 minutes at a time.
1. 5–10 minute naps.
2. None, but alert, aware and looking around.
3. 2–5 minute naps.
4. Less than 2 minute naps. Frequent waking – probably unsettled.
5. None – uneasy and unrestful with it.

Facial expression

Score

0. Eyelids closed and relaxed – no lines, lips slightly apart. No movement of nostrils or face.
1. Eyelids remain closed but face slightly screwed up with lines around mouth, eyes and over brow. Very transient expression and may be repeated often. Baby still asleep but may make mewing noises and sighs with consequent expression.
2. Attentive, receptive expression. Awake and aware and responding to surroundings. Paying interest, no lines on face, slow blinking of eyes. Mouth slowly opening and closing with tongue moving slowly in and out.
3. Eyes partly closed with lines around. Mild furrowing of brow. Face slightly contorted into frown expression. Chin may quiver – gaze be squinted and brow look 'wary'. May be a transient expression throughout assessment.
4. Moderately furrowed brow. Eyes closed and screwed up tightly causing many lines around eyes. Nostrils sharp and flaring. Lips tightly held therefore thin line to mouth when crying. Jutting lower lip may be constant or transient at a ration of 50:50 with either (3) or (5).
5. Practically all the time without relief, a constant deeply furrowed brow. Very flared nostrils, unnaturally open mouth with tightly held lips. Eyes tightly shut. A grey pallor to face.

Liverpool infant distress score chart

NAME:	C/S NO.									D.O.B								DATE:			
ASSESSMENT TIME																					
Spont. movement																					
Spont. excitability																					
Flexion of fingers/toes																					
Tone																					
Cry quantity																					
Cry quality																					
Sleep																					
Facial expression																					
TOTAL SCORE																					
Pulse																					
SaO_2																					
B/P																					
COMMENTS/ANALGESIA																					

REFERENCES

Ambuel, B., Hamlett, K.W., Marx, C.M. & Blumer, J.L. (1992) Assessing distress in pediatric intensive care environments: the COMFORT scale. *Journal of Pediatric Psychology*, **17**, 95–109.

American Academy of Pediatrics (1999) Circumcision policy statement (RE9850). *Pediatrics* **103**, 686–693. Available at www.aap.org, accessed October 2005.

Ansermino, M., Basu, R., Vandebeek, C. & Montgomery, C. (2003) Nonopioid additives to local anaesthetics for caudal blockade in children: a systematic review. *Pediatric Anesthesia* **13** (7), 561–573.

Arana, A., Morton, N.S. & Hansen, T.G. (2001) Treatment with paracetamol in infants. *Acta Anaesthesiologica Scandinavica* **45** (1), 20–29.

Armel, H.E. & Horowitz, M. (1994) Alkalinization of local anaesthesia with sodium bicarbonate – preferred method of local anaesthesia. *Urology* **43**, 101.

Anand, K.J. (2001) Consensus state for the prevention and management of pain in the newborn. *Archives of Pediatric and Adolescent Medicine* **155**, 173–180.

Anand, K.J.S., Shapiro, B.S. & Berde, C.B. (1993) Pharmacotherapy with systemic analgesics. In: Anand, K.J.S. & McGrath, P.J. (eds) *Pain in Neonates*. Elsevier Science, Amsterdam, pp. 155–198.

Blauer, T. & Gertsmann, D. (1998) A simultaneous comparison of three neonatal pain scales during common NICU procedures. *Clinical Journal of Pain* **14**, 39–47.

British National Formulary (2005) *British National Formulary 2005*. Available at www.bnf.org, accessed March 2005.

Bucher, H.U., Baumgartner, N. & Bucher, N. (2000) Artificial sweetener reduces nocioreceptive reaction in term newborn infants. *Early Human Development* **59**, 51–60.

Buchholz, M., Karl, H.W., Pomietto, M. & Lynn, A. (1998) Pain scores in infants: a modified infant pain scale versus visual analogue. *Journal of Pain and Symptom Management* **15**, 117–124.

Buttner, W. & Finke, W. (2002) Analysis of behavioural and physiological parameters for the assessment of postoperative analgesic demand in newborns, infants and young children: a comprehensive report on seven consecutive studies. *Pediatric Anesthesia* **10** (3), 303–318.

Carbajal, R., Puape, A., Hoenn, E., Lenclen, R. & Olivier-Martin, M. (1997) APN: evaluation behavioural scale of acute pain in newborn infants. *Archives of Pediatrics* **4**, 623–628.

Carbajal, R., Veerapen, S. & Couderc, S. (2003) Analgesic effect of breast feeding in term neonates: randomised controlled trial. *British Medical Journal* **326** (7379), 13–15.

Cignacco, E., Mueller, R., Hamers, J.P.H. & Gessler, P. (2004) Pain assessment in the neonate using the Bernese Pain Scale for Neonates. *Early Human Development* **78**, 125–131.

Clark, E.B. (1995) Epidemiology of congenital cardiovascular malformations. In: Emmanouilides, G.C., Allen, H.D., Riemenschneider, T.A. & Gutgesell, H.P. (eds) *Heart Disease in Infants, Children, and Adolescents*, 5th edn. Williams & Wilkins, Baltimore.

Craig, K.D., Whitfield, M.F., Grunau, R.V.E., Linton, J. & Hadjistavropoulos, H.D. (1993) Pain in the preterm neonate: behavioural and physiological indices. *Pain* **52**, 287–299.

Debillon, T., Zupan, V., Ravault, N., Magny, J.-F. & Dehan, M. (2001) Development and initial validation of the EDIN scale, a new tool for assessing prolonged pain in preterm infants. *Archives of Disease in Childhood. Fetal and Neonatal Edition* **85**, F36–F41.

de Wildt, S.N., Kearns, G.L., Hop, W.C.J., Murry, D.J., Abdel-Rahman, S.M. & van den Anker, J.N. (2002) Pharmacokinetics and metabolism of oral midazolam in preterm infants. *British Journal of Clinical Pharmacology* **53** (4), 390–392.

Duhn, L.J. & Medves, J.M. (2004) A systematic integrative review of infant pain assessment tools. *Advanced Neonatal Care* **4** (3), 126–140.

Fanos, V., Benini, D., Verlato, G., Errico, G. & Cuzzolin, L. (2005) Efficacy and renal tolerability of ibuprofen vs. indomethacin in preterm infants with patent ductus arteriosus. *Fundamental and Clinical Pharmacology* **19** (2), 187–193.

Fitzgerald, M. (1993) Development of pain pathways and mechanisms. In: Anand, K.J.S. & McGrath, P.J. (eds) *Pain in Neonates*. Elsevier Science, Amsterdam, pp. 19–37.

Frank, L.S., Cox, S., Allen, A. & Winter, I. (2004) Parental concern and distress about infant pain. *Archives of Disease in Childhood. Fetal and Neonatal Edition* **89**, F71.

Frayling, I.M., Addison, G.M., Chattergee, K. & Meakin, G. (1990) Methaemoglobinaemia in children treated with prilocaine-lignocaine cream. *British Medical Journal* **301**, 153–154.

Friedrichs, J.B., Young, S., Gallagher, D., Keller, C. & Kimura, R.E. (1995) Where does it hurt? An interdisciplinary approach to improving the quality of pain assessment and management in the neonatal intensive care unit. *The Nursing Clinics of North America* **30**, 143–159.

Gallo, A.M. (2003) The fifth vital sign: implementation of the Neonatal Infant Pain Scale. *Journal of Obstetric, Gynecologic and Neonatal Nursing (United States)* **32**, (2), 199–206.

Gaukroger, P.B. (1997) Practical aspects of postoperative analgesia. In: McKenzie, I., Gaukroger, P.B., Ragg, P. & Brown, T.C.K. (Kester) (eds) *Manual of Acute Pain Management in Children*. Churchill Livingstone, New York, pp. 115–119.

Gauvain-Piquard, A., Rodary, C., Rezvani, A. & Lemerle, J. (1987) Pain in children aged 2–6 years: a new observational rating scale elaborated in a pediatric oncology unit – preliminary report. *Pain* **31** (2), 177–188.

Gormally, S., Barr, R.G. & Wertheim, L. (2003) Contact and nutrient caregiving effects on newborn infant pain responses. *Developmental Medicine and Child Neurology* **43**, 28–38.

Gradin, M., Eriksson, M. & Schollin, J. (2002) Pain reduction at venipuncture in newborns: oral glucose compared with local anesthesia. *Pediatrics* **110**, 1053–1057.

Grunau, R.E., Oberlander, T., Holsti, L. & Whitfield, M.F. (1998) Bedside application of the Neonatal Facial Coding System in pain assessment of premature infants. *Pain* **76** (3), 277–286.

Guinsburg, R., Kopelman, B.I., Anand, K.J.S., de Almeida, M.F.B. & de Araujo Peres, C. (1998) Physiological, hormonal and behavioural responses to a single fentanyl dose in intubated and ventilated preterm neonates. *Journal of Pediatrics* **132**, 954–959.

Gunnar, M.R., Fisch, R.O. & Malone, S. (1984) The effects of a pacifying stimulus on behavior and adrenocortical responses to circumcision in the newborn. *Journal of the American Academy of Child and Adolescent Psychiatry* **23**, 34–38.

Hansen, G., O'Brien, K., Morton, N.S. & Rasmussen, S.N. (1999) Plasma paracetamol concentrations and pharmacokinetics following rectal administration in neonates and young infants. *Acta Anaesthesiologica Scandinavica* **43** (8), 855–859.

Hardwick-Smith, S., Mastrobattista, J.M., Wallace, P.A. & Ritchey, M.L. (1998) Ring block for neonatal circumcision. *Obstetrics and Gynecology* **91** (6), 930–934.

Herschel, M., Khoshnood, B., Ellman, C., Maydew, N. & Mittendorf, R. (1998) Neonatal circumcision. Randomized trial of a sucrose pacifier for pain control. *Archives of Pediatric and Adolescent Medicine* **152**, 279–284.

Hodgkinson, K., Bear, M., Thorn, J. & Van Blaricum, S. (1994) Measuring pain in neonates: evaluating an instrument and developing a common language. *Australian Journal of Advanced Nursing* **12**, 17–22.

Horgan, M. & Choonara, I. (1996) Measuring pain in neonates: an objective score. *Pediatric Nursing*, **8**, 24–27.

Howard, C.R., Howard, F.M. & Weitzman, M.L. (1994) Acetaminophen analgesia in neonatal circumcision: the effect on pain. *Pediatrics* **93**, 641–646.

Hudson-Barr, D., Capper-Michel, B., Lambert, S., Palermo, T.M., Morbeto, K. & Lombardo, S. (2002) Validation of the Pain Assessment in Neonates (PAIN) scale with the Neonatal Infant Pain Scale (NIPS). *Neonatal Network* **21** (6), 15–21.

Izard, C.E. (1995) *The Maximally Discriminative Facial Movement Coding System.* University of Delaware, Newark.

Jeffery, H.E., Ius, D. & Page, M. (2000) The role of swallowing during active sleep in the clearance of reflux in term and preterm infants. *Journal of Pediatrics* **137**, 545–548.

Johnston, C.C., Collinge, J.M., Henderson, S.J. & Anand, K.J. (1997) A cross-sectional survey of pain and pharmacological analgesia in

Canadian neonatal intensive care units. *Clinical Journal of Pain* **13**, 308–312.

Joyce, B.A., Schade, J.G., Keck, J.F., Gerkensmeyer, J. & Raftery, T. (1994) Reliability and validity of preverbal pain assessment tools. *Issues in Comprehensive Pediatric Nursing* **17**, 121–135.

Joyce, B.A., Keck, J.F. & Gerkensmeyer, J. (2001) Evaluation of pain management interventions for neonatal circumcision pain. *Journal of Pediatric Health Care* **15**, 105–114.

Koroglu, A., Durmus, M., Togal, T., Ozpolat, Z. & Ersoy, M.O. (2005) Spinal anaesthesia in full-term infants of 0–6 months: are there any differences regarding age? *European Journal of Anaesthesiology* **22** (2), 111–116.

Krechel, S.W. & Bildner, J. (1995) CRIES: a new neonatal postoperative pain measurement score: initial testing of validity and reliability. *Paediatric Anaesthesia* **5**, 53–61.

Kraft, N.L. (2003) A pictorial and video guide to circumcision without pain. *Advanced Neonatal Care* **3** (2), 50–64.

Lander, J., Brady-Fryer, B., Metcalfe, J.B., Nazarali, S. & Muttitt, S. (1997) Comparison of ring block, dorsal penile nerve block, and topical anesthesia for neonatal circumcision: a randomized controlled trial. *JAMA* **278**, 2157–2162.

Lawrence, J., Alcock, D., McGrath, P., Kay, J. & MacMurray, S.B. (1993) The development of a tool to assess neonatal pain. *Neonatal Network* 12, 59–66.

Lesko, S.M. & Mitchell, A.A. (1995) An assessment of the safety of pediatric ibuprofen. A practitioner-based randomized clinical trial. *JAMA* **273**, 929–933.

Lesko, S.A. & Mitchell, A.A. (1999) The safety of acetaminophen and ibuprofen among children younger than two years old. *Pediatrics* **104**, e39.

Levene, M.I. & Quinn, M. (1992) Use of sedatives and muscle relaxants in newborn babies receiving mechanical ventilation. *Archives of Disease in Childhood* **67**, 870–873.

Lin, Yuan-C., Sentivany-Collins, S.K., Peterson, K.L., Boltz, M.G. & Krane, E.J. (1999) Outcomes after single injection caudal epidural versus continuous infusion epidural via caudal approach for postoperative analgesia in infants and children undergoing patent ductus arteriosus ligation. *Pediatric Anesthesia* **9** (2), 139–143.

Loughnan, P. & Ahluwalia, J. (1997) Pain relief in the newborn. In: McKenzie, I., Gaukroger, P.B., Ragg, P. & Brown, T.C.K. (Kester) (eds) *Manual of Acute Pain Management in Children.* Churchill Livingstone, New York, pp. 141–149.

Lucassen, P., Assendelft, W., Gubbels, J.W., van Eijk, M., van Geldrop, W.J. & Knuistingh Neven, A. (1998) Effectiveness of treatments for infantile colic: systematic review. *British Medical Journal* **316** (7144), 1563–1569.

Lugo-Janer, G., Padial, M. & Sanchez, J.L. (1994) Less painful alternatives for local anesthesia. *Journal of Dermatologic Surgery and Oncology* **20**, 155.

Macke, J.K. (2001) Analgesia for circumcision: effects on newborn behaviour and mother/infant interaction. *Journal of Obstetric, Gynecologic and Neonatal Nursing* **30**, 507–514.

Mathew, P.J. & Mathew, J.L. (2003) Assessment and management of pain in infants. *Postgraduate Medical Journal* **79**, 438–443. Available at www.pmj.bmjjournals.com/cgi/content/full/79/934/438.

McCulloch, K.M., Ji, S.A. & Raju, T.N. (1995) Skin blood flow changes during routine nursery procedures. *Early Human Development* **41**, 147–156.

McElhinney, D.B. & Wernovsky, G. (2001) Outcomes of neonates with congenital heart disease. *Current Opinions in Pediatrics* **13**, 104–110.

McGrath, P.J. & Unruh, A.M. (1993) Social and legal issues. In: Anand, K.J.S. & McGrath, P.J. (eds) *Pain in Neonates*. Elsevier Science, Amsterdam, pp. 295–320.

McGrath, P.J., Deveber, L.L. & Hearn, M.T. (1985) Multidimensional pain assessment in children. *Advances in Pain Research and Therapy* **9**, 387–393.

Mohan, C.G., Risucci, D.A., Casimir, M. & Gulrajani-LaCorte, M. (1998) Comparison of analgesics in ameliorating the pain of circumcision. *Journal of Perinatology* **18**, 13–19.

Moore, J. (2001) No more tears: a randomized controlled double-blind trial of amethocaine gel vs placebo in the management of procedural pain in neonates. Issues and innovations in nursing practice. *Journal of Advanced Nursing* **34**, 475–482.

Nandi, R. & Fitzgerald, M. (2005) Opioid analgesia in the newborn. *European Journal of Pain* **9** (2), 105–108.

Pen-Hua, Su, Jia-Yuh, Chen, Chi-Ming, Su, Tzu-Ching, Huang & Hong-Shen, Lee (2003) Comparison of ibuprofen and indomethacin therapy for patent ductus arteriosus in preterm infants. *Pediatrics International* **45** (6), 665–670.

Peters, J.W., Koot, H.M., Grunau, R.E., et al. (2003) Neonatal Facial Coding System for assessing postoperative pain in infants; item reduction is valid and feasible. *Clinical Journal of Pain (United States)* **19** (6), 353–363.

Phillips, P. (1995) Neonatal pain management; a call to action. *Pediatric Nursing* **21** (2), 195–199.

Pokela, M.L. (1994) Pain relief can reduce hypoxemia in distressed neonates during routine treatment procedures. *Pediatrics* **93** (3), 379–383.

Razmus, I.S., Dalton, M.E. & Wilson, D. (2004) Pain management for newborn circumcision. *Pediatric Nursing* **30** (5), 414–417.

Rosenstein, D. & Oster, H. (1988) Differential facial responses for four basic tastes in newborns. *Child Development* **59**, 1555, 1568.

Royal College of Nursing (2005) *The Recognition and Assessment of Acute Pain in Children*. Available at www.rcn.org.uk/publications/pdf/guidelines/cpg_contents.pdf.

Sabrine, N. & Sinha, S. (2000) Pain in neonates. *Lancet* **355**, 932–933.

Schade, J.G., Joyce, B.A., Gerkensmeyer, J. & Keck, J.F. (1996) Comparison of three preverbal scales for postoperative pain assessment in a diverse pediatric sample. *Journal of Pain Symptom Management* **12**, 348–359.

Sparshott, M.M. (1996) The development of a clinical distress scale for ventilated newborn infants: identification of pain and distress based on validated behavioural scores. *Journal of Neonatal Nursing* **2**, 5–11.

Spence, K., Gillies, D., Harrison, D., Johnston, L. & Nagy, S. (2005) A reliable pain assessment tool for clinical assessment in the neonatal intensive care unit. *Journal of Obstetric, Gynecologic and Neonatal Nursing* **34** (1), 80–86.

Stang, H.J. & Snellman, L.W. (1998) Circumcision practice patterns in the United States. *Pediatrics* **101** (6), e5.

Stang, H.J., Gunnar, M.R., Snellman, L., Condon, L.M. & Kestenbaum, R. (1988) Local anesthesia for neonatal circumcision. Effects on distress and cortisol response. *JAMA* **259**, 1507–1511.

Stang, H.J., Snellman, L.W., Condon, L.M., et al. (1997) Beyond dorsal penile nerve block: a more humane circumcision. *Pediatrics* **100** (2), e3.

Sternberg, W.F., Scorr, L., Smith, L.D., Ridgway, C.G. & Stout, M. (2005) Long-term effects of neonatal surgery on adulthood pain behaviour. *Pain* **113** (3), 347–353.

Stevens, B., Johnston, C., Petryshen, P. & Taddio, A. (1996) Premature infant pain profile: development and initial validation. *Clinical Journal of Pain* **12**, 13–22.

Stevens, B., Yamada, J. & Ohlsson, A. (2001) *Sucrose for Analgesia in Newborn Infants Undergoing Painful Procedures*. The Cochrane Library 2001. Available at www.nichd.nih.gov/cochraneneonatal, accessed March 2005.

Stevens, B., McGrath, P., Gibbins, S., et al. (2003) Procedural pain in newborns at risk for neurologic impairment. *Pain* **105**, 1–2, 27–35.

Taddio, A., Nulman, I., Koren, B.S., Stevens, B. & Koren, G. (1995) A revised measure of acute pain in infants. *Journal of Pain and Symptom Management* **10**, 456–463.

Taddio, A., Katz, J., Ilersich, A.L. & Koren, G. (1997a) Effect of neonatal circumcision on pain response during subsequent routine vaccination. *Lancet* **349**, 599–603.

Taddio, A., Stevens, B., Craig, K., et al. (1997b) Efficacy and safety of lidocaine-prilocaine cream for pain during circumcision. *New England Journal of Medicine* **336** (17), 1197–1201.

Taddio, A., Pollock, N., Gilbert-MacLeod, C., Ohlsson, K. & Koren, G. (2000) Combined analgesia and local anesthesia to minimize pain during circumcision. *Archives of Pediatric and Adolescent Medicine* **154**, 620–623.

Taeusch, H.W., Martinez, A.M., Partridge, J.C., Sniderman, S., Armstrong-Wells, J. & Fuentes-Afflick, E. (2002) Pain during Mogen or Plastibell circumcision. *Journal of Perinatology* **22** (3), 214–218.

Tarbell, S.E., Cohen, I.T. & Marsh, J.L. (1992) The Toddler–Preschooler Postoperative Pain Scale: an observational scale for measuring postoperative pain in children aged 1–5. Preliminary report. *Pain* **50**, 273–280.

Tibboel, D., Anand, K.J.S. & van den Anker, J.N. (2005) The pharmacological treatment of neonatal pain. *Seminars in Fetal and Neonatal Medicine* **10** (2), 195–205.

Unruh, A.M. (2002) Pain across the lifespan. In: Strong, J., Unruh, A.M., Wright, A. & Baxter, G.D. (eds) *Pain. A Textbook for Therapists.* Churchill Livingstone, Edinburgh.

Van Dijk, M., Peters, J.W., van Deventer, P., et al. (2005) The Comfort Behaviour Scale: a tool for assessing pain and sedation in infants. *American Journal of Nursing* **105** (1), 33–36.

Weise, K.L. & Nahata, M.C. (2005) EMLA for painful procedures in infants. *Journal of Pediatric Health Care* **19** (1), 42–49.

Williamson, M.L. (1997) Circumcision anesthesia: a study of nursing implications for dorsal penile nerve block. *Pediatric Nursing* **23**, 59–63.

Wolf, R., Doyle, E. & Thomas, E. (1998) Modifying infant stress responses to major surgery: spinal vs extradural vs opioid analgesia. *Pediatric Anesthesia* **8** (4), 305–311.

Woolfson, A.D., McCaffery, D.F. & Boston, V. (1990) Clinical experiences with a novel percutaneous amethocaine preparation: prevention of pain due to venepuncture in children. *British Journal of Clinical Pharmacology* **30**, 273–279.

Zenk, K.E., Sills, J.H. & Koeppel, R.M. (2000) *Neonatal Medications and Nutrition: A Comprehensive Guide*, 2nd edn. NICU Ink, Santa Rosa, California, pp. 288–289.

Pain in Childhood
(6 Months to 12 Years)

4

INTRODUCTION

This chapter considers the special needs of children from 6-month-old infants to 12-year-old adolescents. Like neonates, children have continued to suffer from inadequate pain control. Relatively little is known about the epidemiology of pain in children, as it has not been extensively studied. As Goodman & McGrath (1991) have suggested, reasons for this tolerance might be due to children's pain having little social impact, as it does not result in benefits claimed and days lost from work!

There is relatively little research on children compared with the immense number of studies of adults (see Box 4.1).

LEARNING OBJECTIVES

❏ To understand some of the complexities of managing pain, from toddlers to pre-adolescent children

❏ To identify some of the common causes of toddler and childhood pain

❏ To recognise the special needs that require improved communication and pain assessment in this age group

❏ To explore the interventions that may be appropriate for infants and children

---

Box 4.1 Research on the management of infant pain

Ensuring there is an availability of good research is essential to informing the management of pain in the younger age group, but this has often been neglected. We searched for articles on 'teething' and 'pain'. Our first search using these search words on PubMed Central retrieved one article published in 1978. Another search using 'Science Direct' also found one article concerned about the possibility of seizures following the use of lignocaine in two children, published in 1988. It would appear that studies of pain in some areas in young children are still rare.

ACUTE PAIN

Principles of assessment and evaluation for acute pain

A valid and appropriate pain assessment tool is important as children may not complain or articulate their pain as well as an adult. The selection of a pain assessment tool should be based on the child's preference but must always incorporate a pain scale. Some of the assessment tools mentioned in the previous chapter may be helpful with the pre-verbal child.

The QUESTT pneumonic tool acts as a reminder of the important aspects of pain assessment in children (Baker & Wong 1987):

- **Q**uestion the child
- **U**se pain rating scales
- **E**valuate behaviour and physiological changes
- **S**ecure parents' involvement
- **T**ake the cause of pain into account
- **T**ake action and evaluate results

Examples of pain assessment tools
- **Faces Pain Scale** (from age 3 years). The Faces Pain Scale comprises a set of four to six cartoon-like faces (Bieri et al. 1990).
- **The Wong-Baker FACES Pain Rating scale** (from age 3 years). See Fig. 4.1.
- **The Oucher** (from age 3 years). The Oucher consists of photographs of children in six stages of distress combined with a vertical scale rating the degree of pain (Beyer & Aradine 1986).
- **Poker chip tool** (age 4–8 years). Pain is described as pieces of hurt represented by four poker chips (Hester 1979; Hester et al. 1990):
  — First chip – 'just a little hurt'
  — Second chip – 'a little more hurt'
  — Third chip – 'more hurt'
  — Fourth chip – 'the most hurt you can have'
- **Eland colour scale** (ages 4–10 years). This requires the child to choose coloured pens or crayons and use these to 'colour in pain' within an outline of a child's body using different

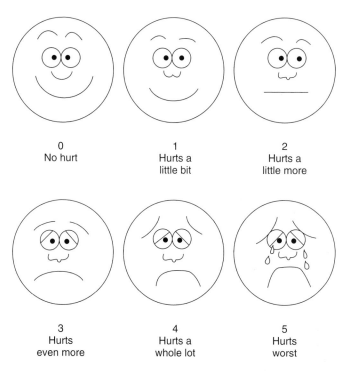

Fig. 4.1 The Wong-Baker FACES Pain Rating Scale. (Reproduced with kind permission from Hockenberry, M.J., Wilson, D. & Winkelstein, M.L. (2005) *Wong's Essentials of Pediatric Nursing*, 7th edn, p. 1259. Mosby, St. Louis. Used with permission. Copyright, Mosby.)

colours, red representing pain and cooler colours less pain (Eland 1985).

- **Derbyshire Children's Hospital pain tool** (ages 6–12 years). This tool uses facial expression, body movement and verbal expression (Peden et al. 2005).
- **Visual analogue scale** (ages 9–10 years). See Fig. 1.3.
- **Pain Assessment Tool for Children (PATCH)** (all ages). PATCH has been developed for use with all children (Qureshi & Buckingham 1994).

- **Child/Parent Total Quality Pain Management (TQPM) instrument** (suitable for children aged 3+). TQPM was developed to provide a standardised instrument to measure quality improvements in the management of pain for children following surgery (Foster & Varni 2002).
- **Waldron/Varni Pediatric Pain Coping Inventory** (suitable for children aged 3+). This was developed to standardise the assessment of children's individual pain coping strategies to help the understanding of individual differences in children's pain reports and perceptions (Varni et al. 1996).
- **Paediatric Pain Profile (PPP)** (suitable for children aged 3+). PPP is a behaviour rating scale for assessing pain in children with severe physical and learning impairments. By necessity it is quite a complex tool but comes with full instructions and is downloadable from the Internet. See www.ppprofile.org.uk (accessed September 2005).

Resources

- Royal College of Paediatrics and Child Health, *Guidelines for Good Practice. The Recognition and Assessment of Acute Pain in Children.* See www.rcpch.ac. uk/publications/clinical_docs/acute_pain.pdf (accessed September 2005)
- Royal College of Nursing, *Clinical Practice Guidelines. The Recognition and Assessment of Acute Pain in Children.* See www.rcn.org.uk/publications/pdf/ guidelines/cpg_contents.pdf (accessed September 2005)
- Institute of Child Health, Great Ormond Street Hospital, *Children's Pain Assessment Project.* See www.ich.ucl.ac.uk/cpap

---

Physiological changes

Acute pain is all part of growing up, but we know that neurological changes take place when humans are exposed to pain. What children experience in terms of pain and suffering and its impact on and the responses of those around them have long-term effects on a child's future pain perception. The responses of adults to pain are shaped by their own upbringing and the way their parents responded to their pain, as revealed in the differing family responses in the case study below.

Case study

At play group the staff notice that when Edward, who is 18 months old, falls over he usually does not cry. He is the fourth boy in a very robust and busy family. Conversely Julian, who is the same age, cries easily and the slightest bump can be a dramatic event. Julian was born a month prematurely and has always been a very precious only child for Derek and Liz.

Children whose pain is closely attended to may respond differently, as adults, to those who have grown up in a more 'rough and tumble' family.

Teething

A child's first teeth usually start to erupt from about 6 months; though often described as 'cutting' new teeth, it is the chemical signals between the cells in the gums that cause some cells to selectively die and separate, allowing the teeth to push through. The process of teething can still be uncomfortable because of movement and changes in the jawbone. Common teething symptoms may be:

- General irritability
- Poor sleeping
- Drooling
- Chewing on everything
- Problems feeding
- Flushed cheeks
- Diarrhoea
- Nappy rash

Any pain should be short-lived and stop as a new tooth appears. Pyrexia is not a feature of teething and may warrant further investigation.

Pharmacological strategies
Paracetamol or ibuprofen syrup can be very helpful, especially at night if discomfort is causing sleeplessness. Rubbing the baby's

gums with a local anaesthetic gel available over the counter at a pharmacy may also be helpful.

Non-pharmacological strategies
- Massaging the baby's gums, using a wet finger
- Giving the baby hard foods such as crusts and rusks to chew on
- Cold teething rings

Surgery
The following are examples of common procedures for infants and children:

- Circumcision
- Appendicectomy
- Thoracotomy for congenital defect
- Hypospadias repair (surgery on male infants to reposition the urethra when it does not exit at the tip of the penis)
- Laparotomy for ureteric reimplantation, pyeloplasty
- Inguinal hernia repair, hydrocele, orchiopexy
- Umbilical hernia repair
- Ventilating ear tubes, antral washout, adenoidectomy
- Tonsillectomy
- Second stage cleft palate surgery
- Squint surgery

Experiencing postoperative pain (short stay)
If children are going to be discharged within hours of surgery, safe and effective pain control must be provided. Children and their parents will need to be informed about how to manage pain, what to look for, what to expect and how to keep pain under control. Once a child is in pain, significantly more analgesia will be required to re-establish pain control and it is likely that he or she will be anxious and frightened. This has implications for future health experiences. Effective early analgesia will reduce the risk of 'wind up'. Children's pain needs to be actively managed, as they may not ask for analgesia. Oral medication is best for children, but the intravenous (IV) route can be used for rapid titration whilst in hospital. Intramuscular injections should never be given and the rectal route is unacceptable for many children.

> **Case study**
>
> Peter aged 9 came to the Day Case Unit for an elective tonsillectomy. He had had a bad experience during previous minor surgery and was very distressed for at least 24 hours afterwards. His parents felt his pain control was inadequate but said nobody took their concerns seriously, with the staff just saying the pain would soon go.

We know that tonsillectomy is very painful, although fortunately most children appear to experience less pain than adults undergoing the same procedure (Graumuller & Laudien 2003). Romsing et al. (1998) studied children receiving both regular and *pro re nata* (prn) paracetamol at recommended therapeutic doses for the first three days after discharge. They found that the prevalence of pain amongst all the children was high, with up to 64% rating their pain as severe despite being on regular medication. Romsing et al. in 2000 looked to see if pain control could be improved by substituting paracetamol for diclofenac but found that pain scores in both groups remained high. They also found that the incidence of nausea and/or vomiting increased with pain and this can be a factor in delaying discharge. Adequate control of pain can not only reduce the distress of children and their families but also result in earlier discharge and reduced costs for the hospital.

Pharmacological strategies
It may well be that for significant numbers of children the pain of tonsillectomy will only be adequately controlled when a range of pharmacological strategies are offered together by combining local anaesthetics with non-opioids and opioids. Health care professionals tend to shy away from strong opioids for children and offer them just codeine or an alternative weak opioid. Our experience suggests that small doses of oral morphine syrup combined with paracetamol and/or an NSAID can be very effective.

To confirm this, we found that studies looking at codeine and paracetamol given to children following tonsillectomy suggest that analgesia was less than adequate (Sutters et al. 2004).

Codeine increases the problems of nausea, emesis and constipation (Moir et al. 2000), and for pain that is still present after a full dose of paracetamol and an NSAID the benefit may not be worth the increased side effects. However, more research is needed.

Oral morphine solution is easily swallowed and the analgesia it can provide promotes the early intake of food and drink. Early oral intake can reduce the risk of slough building up on the tonsil beds, thereby reducing the risk of infection and subsequent postoperative bleeding. We do know that NSAIDs have an effect on blood clotting time and are therefore sometimes associated with an increased bleeding risk. Some studies have not found this to be a problem when NSAIDs are used postoperatively (Romsing et al. 2000), and it may be that their pre-emptive use only may contribute to bleeding (Schmidt et al. 2001). There is little doubt that local anaesthetics are probably underutilised, with recent studies illustrating benefits (Kaygusuz & Susaman 2003; Somdas et al. 2004).

Non-pharmacological strategies
Reducing anxiety and anticipated pain through parental knowledge and involvement can be helpful as well as ensuring the child feels he or she will be believed when reporting pain. Early activity and sending a child home to a familiar environment as soon as possible may also help to reduce the perception of pain. Bringing in favourite toys or bedding perhaps provides a familiar and comforting environment. Many hospitals encourage parents to stay with their children and even accompany them to the anaesthetic room.

Experiencing postoperative pain (longer stay)

Case study

Mary aged 5 returns to the ward following a laparotomy to reimplant her ureters. She has an epidural in situ and her parents are delighted to find her completely pain free in recovery. The staff in the paediatric unit are very experienced and undertake regular pain assessment and monitoring to ensure she remains pain free. They continue with pain assessment involving the parents once the epidural is discontinued and Mary makes a rapid and complication-free recovery.

This case study represents a positive example of how pain can be well managed.

Pharmacological strategies

Once the more 'high tech' approaches to postoperative pain management such as epidurals and patient controlled analgesia (PCA) are discontinued the control of pain may still require regular oral analgesia until the child is pain free. Acute pain is relatively easy to manage in children and the algorithm shown in Fig. 4.2 may provide a useful reminder of an effective strategy for most acute pain and can be placed in a prominent place within the children's ward.

The basic principles of acute pain control always include using local anaesthetic drugs intraoperatively when and where possible, and an epidural is an excellent example of how a combination of local anaesthetic and an opioid such as fentanyl can provide complete postoperative analgesia at rest.

If an epidural is not possible, use paracetamol as a routine analgesia with a loading dose of either oral 20 mg/kg prior to surgery or rectal 30 g/kg following induction of analgesia, then reverting to 10–15 mg/kg on a regular basis until pain subsides. Other analgesics such as NSAIDs and opioids can be added as needed, taking advantage of the synergistic effect of balanced analgesia. These drugs may still be required for a period of time once an epidural has been discontinued to ensure children remain as pain free as possible into their recovery period.

Consider the use of a sticky label for prescribed analgesics that can be adhered to the prescription charts of children with acute pain. This may reduce the risk of error and can be popular with staff, patients and their parents as delays in prescribing are minimised. A sticker may also encourage the use of effective multimodal analgesia, which is often overlooked in children. It also enables any postoperative opioid-related nausea and vomiting to be rapidly treated with an antiemetic (in the case of Fig. 4.3, ondansetron).

Without adequate pain control the risks for children may be just as serious as for adults, resulting in:

- Respiratory complications
- Stress-related catabolic states

- Immunosuppression
- Neurological pain ('wind up')
- Psychological stress
- Loss of confidence in hospital staff
- Fear of any future intervention
- Reluctance to report pain if previously ignored

Specific issues in the operating theatre include raising the profile of paediatric pain control and addressing parental accompanying rights in the recovery area and at anaesthesia induction. Having specially trained children's nurses available in recovery can also help to improve communications and pain control.

Pharmacological strategies for managing specific postoperative pain

Inguinal hernia repair or orchiopexy
Doctors should consider giving paracetamol regularly following a loading dose, wound infiltration or an ileoinguinal block or 1 ml/kg of caudal bupivacaine 0.25% plus regular paracetamol and/or ibuprofen for at least 24 hours. Titrated oral morphine syrup or a comparable opioid should still be available for any breakthrough pain.

Open appendicectomy
This is less common these days as appendicectomies can be conducted via a laparoscope. Consider paracetamol with a loading dose plus an IV opioid such as morphine intraoperatively and wound infiltration with local anaesthetic. Employ PCA for postoperative pain management until the child is eating and drinking well. PCA can be used with children of more or less any age as long as they can understand the concept and press the button appropriately. Consider continuing with regular paracetamol and/or ibuprofen for at least 24 hours postoperatively or from the time the PCA is discontinued.

Lacerations, foreign bodies and abscesses
Give paracetamol with a loading dose and then on a regular basis postoperatively for the first day, and then as needed. Consider wound infiltration with 0.25% bupivacaine.

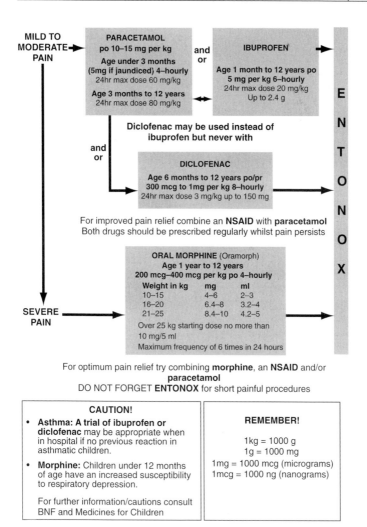

MILD TO MODERATE PAIN

PARACETAMOL
po 10–15 mg per kg

Age under 3 months
(5mg if jaundiced) 4–hourly
24hr max dose 60 mg/kg

Age 3 months to 12 years
24hr max dose 80 mg/kg

and or

IBUPROFEN

Age 1 month to 12 years po
5 mg per kg 6–hourly
24hr max dose 20 mg/kg
Up to 2.4 g

Diclofenac may be used instead of
ibuprofen but never with

and or

DICLOFENAC

Age 6 months to 12 years po/pr
300 mcg to 1mg per kg 8–hourly
24hr max dose 3 mg/kg up to 150 mg

For improved pain relief combine an **NSAID** with **paracetamol**
Both drugs should be prescribed regularly whilst pain persists

ORAL MORPHINE (Oramorph)
Age 1 year to 12 years
200 mcg–400 mcg per kg po 4–hourly

Weight in kg	mg	ml
10–15	4–6	2–3
16–20	6.4–8	3.2–4
21–25	8.4–10	4.2–5

Over 25 kg starting dose no more than
10 mg/5 ml
Maximum frequency of 6 times in 24 hours

SEVERE PAIN

E N T O N O X

For optimum pain relief try combining **morphine**, an **NSAID** and/or
paracetamol
DO NOT FORGET **ENTONOX** for short painful procedures

CAUTION!

- **Asthma: A trial of ibuprofen or diclofenac** may be appropriate when in hospital if no previous reaction in asthmatic children.

- **Morphine:** Children under 12 months of age have an increased susceptibility to respiratory depression.

  For further information/cautions consult BNF and Medicines for Children

REMEMBER!

1kg = 1000 g
1g = 1000 mg
1mg = 1000 mcg (micrograms)
1mcg = 1000 ng (nanograms)

Fig. 4.2 A pain management algorithm designed to promote effective pain control using multimodal therapy in children (dosages taken from Royal College of Paediatrics and Child Health 1999). (Reproduced with kind permission of Poole Hospital NHS Trust where the algorithm has been used effectively since 1999.)

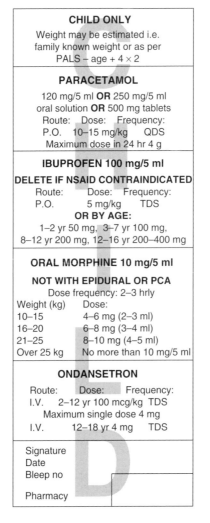

> **CHILD ONLY**
> Weight may be estimated i.e.
> family known weight or as per
> PALS – age + 4 × 2
>
> **PARACETAMOL**
> 120 mg/5 ml **OR** 250 mg/5 ml
> oral solution **OR** 500 mg tablets
> Route: Dose: Frequency:
> P.O.   10–15 mg/kg   QDS
> Maximum dose in 24 hr 4 g
>
> **IBUPROFEN 100 mg/5 ml**
> **DELETE IF NSAID CONTRAINDICATED**
> Route: Dose: Frequency:
> P.O.   5 mg/kg   TDS
> **OR BY AGE:**
> 1–2 yr 50 mg, 3–7 yr 100 mg,
> 8–12 yr 200 mg, 12–16 yr 200–400 mg
>
> **ORAL MORPHINE 10 mg/5 ml**
> **NOT WITH EPIDURAL OR PCA**
> Dose frequency: 2–3 hrly
> Weight (kg)   Dose:
> 10–15   4–6 mg (2–3 ml)
> 16–20   6–8 mg (3–4 ml)
> 21–25   8–10 mg (4–5 ml)
> Over 25 kg   No more than 10 mg/5 ml
>
> **ONDANSETRON**
> Route: Dose: Frequency:
> I.V.   2–12 yr 100 mcg/kg TDS
> Maximum single dose 4 mg
> I.V.   12–18 yr 4 mg   TDS
>
> Signature
> Date
> Bleep no
>
> Pharmacy

Fig. 4.3 Paediatric analgesia sticker which can be placed on the prescribing chart to reduce error and help to promote effective analgesia. (Reproduced with kind permission of Poole Hospital NHS Trust.)

Thoracotomy
Doctors should ideally consider an epidural infusion or a loading dose of a strong opioid such as morphine or fentanyl intraoperatively. Use intercostal blocks, or PCA or NCA (nurse controlled analgesia) if blocks fail or are not used or the epidural fails. Continue with paracetamol regularly until the child is pain free.

Lower limb surgery
Give a loading dose of paracetamol, plus regular doses for at least two days postoperatively. PCA and/or femoral or sciatic nerve blocks can be used, but caution is needed and close monitoring required for compartment syndrome.

Non-pharmacological strategies
• Simple comforting and reassurance can be very effective for children
• Stroking the child's head and holding them close may be helpful
• Distraction appears to be more effective in children than it is for adults. Examples include reading stories, drawing, the television, 'gameboy' computer games and particularly virtual reality computer games (see Box 4.2 later in the text associated with managing trauma pain).

Resources

• Huth et al. (2004) for information on imagery following surgery
• Jylli et al. (2002) for information on epidural analgesia
• Peters et al. (1999) for information on PCA analgesia
• Pölkki et al. (2001) for information on non-pharmacological strategies
• Pölkki et al. (2003) for a study of children's hospital experiences

Trauma
Some common causes of trauma in this age group are as follows:

• Road traffic accidents
• Fractures
• Burns and scalds
• Lacerations
• Foreign bodies

Experiencing acute trauma pain

Case study

Peter is 7 years old and has had to be admitted to hospital to immobilise a badly fractured tibia and fibula. He may face surgery or a period of traction and his parents are very concerned and distressed about how his pain will be controlled because at the moment he is yelling and screaming and they feel very shocked. Peter is picking up on their distress and is proving a challenge to nurses in the Accident and Emergency Department.

In the Accident and Emergency Department ensure a valid pain assessment tool is used as soon as possible. The Wong-Baker FACES Pain Rating Scale (see Fig. 4.1) and/or a numerical rating scale (0 to 10 or 0 to 5; see Fig. 1.5) may be the most appropriate as they are quick and easy to use. Consider altering documentation to incorporate a pain score on all observation charts and clinical pathways. Also consider the implementation of IV opioid bolus administration by nurses who have undertaken a training and competency package for children whose pain is inadequately controlled by first-line non-opioid therapy. Clinical decision-making guidelines can be developed to improve the consistency of identifying and managing problems associated with pain management in children immediately the child arrives in the Accident and Emergency Department. Patient group directives that are popular for adult care pathways can also be developed to assist nurses to manage children's pain rapidly in an emergency department. Pain assessment that is incorporated into routine care will reassure parents that pain is a priority and hopefully allay their fears and anxieties. It will also ensure that any analgesics that are given are evaluated for their effectiveness or potential side effects.

Communication between clinical teams regarding interventions that are effective and those that are not will ensure that only strategies that have been beneficial are continued. At all stages include the parents in the assessment procedure, as they will often be the first to recognise pain rather than distress in their child. Parents will need considerable support to ensure they do not alarm and frighten their child because their fears and anxieties may be easily transferred to their child. Calm reassurance can go a long way to pacifying a frightened child and an anxious parent.

Pharmacological strategies
Intranasal diamorphine may be especially useful when rapid pain relief is needed and intravenous access is difficult or will not be required. It can be far less traumatic than anything that involves a needle (Wilson et al. 1997; Davies & Crawford 2001).

Fractures
Fractures requiring surgery will need strong opioids preoperatively and intraoperatively plus a loading dose of paracetamol and then regular paracetamol doses for at least two days. Nerve blocks given as a single injection or maintained with a catheter can be very effective for a major bone fracture such as a femur in adults (Stella et al. 2000), but there is little published research on the use of this effective technique in children under 14 years old.

Burns and scalds
These invariably require painful dressing changes and debridement as well as immediate pain relief during the acute stage. Effective strategies for ongoing pain may include continuous opioid infusions, PCA, NCA, regular oral opioids, paracetamol and/or ibuprofen. If skin grafting is required then a nerve block to the donor site may also be needed, as these sites can be very painful. For dressing changes consider premedication with oral midazolam and the use of Entonox. Intravenous conscious sedation using such combinations as midazolam and an opioid such as alfentanyl or an analgesic/anaesthetic agent such as ketamine supervised by an anaesthetist or suitably qualified professional can be extremely effective. In some cases, however, the pain of a dressing change may require a general anaesthetic.

Lacerations
Follow the basic guidelines of multimodal analgesia including topical anaesthesia either alone or prior to infiltration with local

anaesthetic. Nerve blocks can be very effective. Using wound glue will be less traumatic than stitching. Consider sedation or even general anaesthesia for suturing major lacerations. Intranasal diamorphine or fentanyl can also be very useful and avoids the added trauma of a needle stick if IV drugs are not necessary.

Foreign bodies
Foreign bodies in children are usually extracted from the nose or the ear and their removal is reported to be more successful following sedation only (Brown et al. 2004). It is unlikely that children will require any analgesia for the procedure, although the removal of foreign bodies from the nose in particular may be uncomfortable.

Non-pharmacological strategies
There is a limit to the effectiveness of any one therapy; however, the effects of two or more therapies given in conjunction are cumulative (Jay et al. 1985). With the exception of cold, which can be used effectively to help reduce pain in all age groups, non-pharmacological strategies such as distraction and relaxation can only dull the perception of pain to make it more tolerable, not necessarily less severe in its intensity (Twycross 1998).

Distraction
Distraction can be a particularly effective strategy when used with children for brief episodes of procedural pain, but the strategy needs to interest the child and be appropriate to his or her level of concentration. Ideally the distraction should stimulate the major sensory pathways of hearing, vision, touch and movement. Examples include holding a favourite soft toy, singing, games and puzzles, describing imaginary journeys, blowing air bubbles, reading pop-up books, looking through kaleidoscopes or viewers, watching television and especially playing interactive and virtual reality computer games if age and development permits (see Box 4.2).

Touch
The need to be touched is present at birth and is a powerful way to communicate caring. Unfortunately for children in hospital

---

Box 4.2 The benefits of virtual reality games for pain management

Contemporary studies are providing strong evidence that virtual reality-based games can greatly enhance analgesia with minimal side effects and little impact on the physical hospital environment. Pain is always experienced as a complex mix of sensory and emotional experience. Distraction, especially in the absorbing format of virtual reality games, can have a positive and measurable impact on the intensity and 'unpleasantness' of pain perceived by children undergoing venepuncture and painful burns dressings (Hoffman et al. 2000, 2004; Hunter et al. 2004; Gold et al. 2005; Kim et al. 2005).

---

they may only experience touch from health care professionals when it is associated with physical examinations or undertaking procedures (Mitchell 1985). Encouraging parents to stroke their child or having another health care professional available to stroke a child's forehead whilst distracting the child with other means can be helpful.

Cognitive strategies

These include helping children understand what is going on and giving them a sense of involvement and control. Ensuring that children do not construe pain or painful procedures as a punishment is important. Warn them that a procedure is likely to be painful but explain the need for it and that together you are going to do everything you can to make the pain bearable. The following gives a synopsis of the strategies that may help to reduce anxiety and thus decrease pain:

• Giving children information in a way they can understand
• Letting them handle any equipment
• Enabling children to practise the procedure themselves on a doll or teddy bear
• Introducing children to all the staff who will be closely involved in their care
• Discussing fears, feelings and any strategies you are going to use together with children and their parents so that they feel part of the procedure and not just a victim of it

Hypnotherapy

This has been used successfully in children who have to undergo painful procedures associated with cancer treatments (Zelter &

LeBaron 1982), but not many clinicians have the skills to offer this as a complementary therapy.

Cognitive-behavioural strategies
- Desensitisation – gradual exposure to the things that frighten and hurt. Positive reinforcement gives the child a meaningful reward for effective coping strategies
- Thought-stopping, where a child can recite a clear positive statement when he or she starts thinking about a dreaded procedure
- Attention-distraction, where a child focuses on breathing exercises during the procedure
- Imagery and fantasy woven into the medical situation

A checklist mnemonic can help focus on the specific issues that can be helpful in preparing a child for a potentially painful procedure, e.g. NITPIC (adapted from Twycross 1998) (see Box 4.3).

Box 4.3 The NITPIC checklist

- **Needs** to be told things, listened to, reassured, respected, offered coping strategies and an assessment of his or her resources
- **Interventions** including pharmacological, non-pharmacological and psychological
- **Time** planning, discussion, interventions and feedback
- **Plan** available resources, strategies and a framework
- **Involve** parents, siblings, medical staff and other appropriate professionals
- **Communicate** with the child, family, siblings, within the team and between colleagues in order to deal with anxiety in the child and his or her parents

---

Resources

- Borland et al. (2002) for information on intranasal fentanyl
- Finley & McGrath (2001) for information on acute and procedural pain
- Franck & Jones (2003) for information on computer-taught coping skills
- Wilson et al. (1997) and Davies & Crawford (2001) for information on intranasal diamorphine

Musculoskeletal or body wall pain

Kim (2002) provides a useful resource on musculoskeletal pain in adolescents and points out that diagnostic criteria are different for this age group, compared to those used in adults.

Back pain

In this age group back pain is particularly common and possibly associated with carrying heavy school bags, although the evidence does not currently support this. There is, however, evidence that children with low back pain are more likely to have negative psychosocial experiences, are more likely to complain of other musculoskeletal pain or have hypermobility. (See *PRODIGY Guidance, Back Pain – Lower*, www.prodigy.nhs.uk/guidance.asp?gt=back%20pain%20-%20lower, accessed October 2005) Posture is also thought to be associated with back pain (Murphy et al. 2004).

Regular paracetamol for a few days should be sufficient and both parents and the child should be educated on the importance of activity and exercise. Being taught how to carry bags with the least strain should improve the situation if school bags are still thought to be a cause of the problem. Serious underlying disorders are uncommon in children; however, despite this, studies of low back pain in children have demonstrated that disability is frequently reported (Salminen et al. 1992). Perhaps more importantly, adolescent experiences of low back pain may herald the onset of intermittent or chronic trouble in adulthood (Olsen et al. 1992; Harreby et al. 1995).

Parapatellar knee pain syndrome or chondromalacia patellae

The cause is unknown but the knee pain is made worse by activities such as running, jumping, doing knee bends or sitting for a long time. Treatment consists of rest from any activity that regularly makes the pain worse, strengthening exercises and using an anti-inflammatory such as ibuprofen.

Slipped capital femoral epiphysis

This is caused by a fracture of the growth plate and slippage of the femoral epiphysis off the femoral neck. Treatment usually requires pinning of the joint and regular non-opioids, with opioids if required for postoperative pain relief.

Osgood-Schlatter disease

This is associated with a tender lump near the top of the tibia. Specific treatment is not usually required other than reassurance and protection of the tender area with a kneepad. The pain resolves spontaneously (after 1–2 years) as the bones complete their growth.

Osteochondritis dissecans

This is caused by formation of a fragment of bone. The knee is the most common site but it may also occur in the elbow or ankle. Minor cases may resolve spontaneously, but older children may require regular non-opioid analgesia and arthroscopic surgery.

Patellar dislocation

This is common in athletes but can also occur in non-athletic individuals. It is treated by immobilisation for 6 weeks, regular non-opioid analgesia for as long as required and quadricep strengthening exercises. In some cases surgery may be necessary but usually a conservative approach is sufficient.

Costochondritis

Costochondritis may be associated with a mild respiratory infection or develop following exercise and is more common in girls. The pain is sometimes made worse by breathing and the discomfort may radiate to the chest, back or abdomen. There is tenderness in the middle of the chest directly over the breastbone. It can be treated with heat and regular over-the-counter pain medication such as paracetamol or ibuprofen.

Benign hypermobility

Children or young adults with hypermobility usually have joint pain or mild swelling during the evening or after exercise. The pain is more common in the lower extremities, such as the calf or thigh muscles, and most often involves large joints such as the knees or elbows. Regular paracetamol may be more useful than an NSAID. Strengthening and balancing exercises are important to reduce flexibility and increase muscle strength to help prevent injury. In addition, children should avoid sitting cross-legged, try wearing shoes with good arch supports and be encouraged not to entertain friends by contorting into interesting stances or 'popping' their joints! Avoiding excessive weight gain and braces or taping may also help to protect affected joints during activities.

Growing pains

These are normal and are experienced in about 25–40% of children. They are more likely to occur in early childhood between the ages of 3 and 5 years or later between 8 and 12 years. There is no specific evidence that bone growth is the cause and children normally experience aches after increased activity during the day. Pain is mostly felt in the muscles of the thighs and calves rather than in joints and children respond well to reassurance, massage, warmth, movement and a cuddle. Some children may occasionally require paracetamol or ibuprofen if pain is problematic at night, but growing pains are rarely experienced every day and resolve spontaneously.

Visceral pain

For most visceral pain, treatment should be directed at the underlying cause following diagnosis, aided by repeated physical examination, undertaken by the same physician over a period of time (Scholer et al. 1999). Traditionally, the use of analgesics has been discouraged in children with abdominal pain for fear of interfering with accurate evaluation and diagnosis. However, several prospective, randomised studies have shown that analgesics may actually enhance diagnostic accuracy by permitting detailed examination of a more cooperative patient (Zoltie & Cust 1986; Attard et al. 1992; Pace & Burke 1996).

The following acute pains will require immediate treatment to rectify the condition in addition to adequate pain relief, including the use of strong opioids for some of the most painful conditions.

Infection

Infection is caused by ingesting contaminated food or water and is associated with painful diarrhoea and vomiting. It usually resolves rapidly and spontaneously once the contaminant has been ejected and the infection brought under control with antibiotics if appropriate. Analgesia is not usually given for this unpleasant but spasmodic pain. Comfort and warmth may help.

Hepatitis

As most drugs are metabolised by the liver, analgesia to combat the pain associated with hepatitis will have to be given with great care, dosages reduced and children carefully monitored.

Ruptured spleen

This can cause major bleeding with severe pain. Treatment will usually involve surgery to remove the spleen and the child should be treated postoperatively with balanced analgesia as for any other major upper abdominal surgery.

Urinary tract infections

These occur in about 3% of girls and 1% of boys by age 11, with symptoms ranging from slight burning with urination and unusual smelling urine to severe pain and high fever. Treatment is usually rapid and effective with appropriate antibiotics. The pain is difficult to treat as it is usually associated with just background loin or bladder pain but with severe discomfort only during urination. Keeping the urine dilute by drinking plenty of clear fluid may make voiding slightly less painful.

Testicular torsion

This can occur if a testis twists, blocking blood flow to the spermatic cord. Once this happens a testis is likely to become damaged and 'die' unless its blood flow is quickly restored by surgery performed within 6 hours. It typically occurs in teenage boys shortly after puberty but can also occur in newborn babies. The principal symptom is severe pain that develops quickly in the affected testis, but it may also be felt in the middle of the abdomen. The pain may require strong multimodal analgesia until surgery can be performed as an emergency.

The following is a list of chronic conditions that may cause an acute flair of visceral pain but rarely lead to pain experienced all the time.

- **Lactose intolerance.** Lactose intolerance is the name given to difficulty digesting the lactose sugar in milk. Pain can only be treated by dietary changes.
- **Mesenteric lymphadenitis.** This is a common cause of right iliac fossa pain in children and is often mistaken for appendicitis. It is usually due to non-specific inflammation of the mesenteric lymph nodes, which causes pain in the terminal ileum. Pain relief includes the usual strategies of regular paracetamol and/or an NSAID, but the pain may sometimes be severe enough to require a strong opioid for a short period, as the condition is self-limiting.
- **Constipation.** It is extremely important to treat this problem. Usually a change in diet to increase fibre intake by consuming more pulses, nuts, grains, fruit and vegetables and plenty of non-sugary fluids will be sufficient. Certain fruits, including papaya and cantaloupe, are very high in fibre and popcorn may be an acceptable and effective way of increasing fibre intake in children over 5 years of age. Some children may need a mild laxative such as lactulose (Cephulac) for a short period. Opioids will always make this problem worse.

Resources

- Royal Children's Hospital, Melbourne, Anaesthesia and Pain Management, Children's Pain Management Service. See www.rch.org.au/anaes/pain/index.cfm?doc_id=781
- For information on acute pain management the following may be useful: McKenzie et al. (1997); Twycross et al. (1997); Morton (1998)

CHRONIC PAIN

Chronic pain is a significant but underrecognised problem in the paediatric population and has been estimated to affect 15–20% of children (Goodman & McGrath 1991). There are many types of chronic pain that children can experience, for example, pain caused by diseases such as cancer, arthritis, sickle cell anaemia, haemophilia, neuralgia, accidental trauma, HIV infection and burns. Most children who have chronic or recurrent types of pain cope quite well. There is, however, a small group of children whose lives become significantly disrupted because of chronic pain. An inability to cope with pain may lead to disability (Dangel 2005). The emotional and social impacts of pain and disability can have far reaching effects on children and their families. There may also be an additional financial burden in terms of reduced working opportunities for the parents. The physical and psychological consequences associated with chronic pain may predispose them to the development of adult chronic pain (Walker et al. 1995). The most important activity is a comprehensive assessment and then appropriate interventions can be selected to meet the needs of the child and his or her family.

Principles of assessment and evaluation for chronic pain

The assessment of chronic pain is essential for the development and evaluation of an individual plan of care specific to each child which takes into consideration his or her pain complaint, intellectual and physical development, comprehension and individual preference. This will need to look at the many facets of chronic pain and its effect on the child's enjoyment of life, ability to interact with friends and family, and schooling as well as the impact pain has on his or her sleep and other activities of living.

Examples of pain assessment tools
Finley & McGrath (1997) is an excellent resource as an in depth guide to the measurement and assessment of pain in infants and children.

- **Adolescent Paediatric Pain Tool (APPT)** is described for use in postoperative pain but can be a useful tool for chronic pain as well (Savedra et al. 1993).
- **Paediatric Pain Profile (PPP)** is a behaviour rating scale for assessing pain in children with severe physical and learning impairments. See www.ppprofile.org.uk (accessed September 2005)
- **Varni-Thompson Questionnaire.** See Varni et al. (1987).
- **Diaries.** These can be simple paper diaries as used by adults, or perhaps more likely to appeal to children are electronic diaries (Palermo et al. 2004a).
- **Child Activity Limitations Interview.** This has been developed to assess recurrent pain in childhood and how this

impacts on children's everyday functioning and daily activities. In particular, the tool can be used to identify appropriate targets for intervention and measure response to such interventions (Palermo et al. 2004a).

Neuropathic pain

Sources of chronic neuropathic pain that may be seen in children are listed below.

Type 1 diabetes

A subclinical neuropathy is common but rarely painful in children (Meh & Denislic 1998). See Chapter 6 and the section on 'Experiencing neuropathic pain' in adults.

Complex regional pain syndrome type 1 (CRPS 1)

Previously known as reflex sympathetic dystrophy CRPS 1 is often not recognised in children. As in adults, this pain may develop following often a relatively minor injury. It is not limited to the distribution of a single peripheral nerve and pain is disproportionate to the severity of the initial injury or tissue damage. It may be associated with some or all of the following:

- Temperature changes in the affected area
- Changes in skin blood flow and sweating
- Oedema
- Bruising
- Allodynia (pain caused by usually non-painful stimuli such as stroking the skin)
- Hyperalgesia (increased sensitivity to painful stimuli)
- Trophic changes such as muscle wasting, loss of hair, shiny parchment-like skin and joint stiffness
- Bone density may decrease and limb shortening occur if the condition becomes long standing

The child will be very protective of the limb or affected area and may describe the pain as burning, aching, throbbing or lancinating. In children the condition is more commonly seen in girls, with lower limbs more often affected, and it may possibly be associated with children who strive to achieve (Walker & Eyres 1997). Early diagnosis is the key to improvement, but unfortunately the average time to diagnosis has been reported to be one year (Wilder et al. 1992).

Pharmacological strategies
- Minimise nociception from any underlying injury with simple analgesia and/or opioids. Analgesia alone, however, is rarely effective for CRPS 1. An IV opioid trial with alfentanyl is probably the best way to test for opioid responsiveness, but the general consensus is that strong opioids for children are usually best avoided for this particular condition if possible (McGrath & Finley 1999).
- Early sympathetic nerve block with a local anaesthetic may help confirm diagnosis, but more research is needed.
- Guanathidine block at an early stage appears to be more effective in children than adults, but as it is done under general anaesthesia this may have an influence on the outcome (Olsson & Berde 1993).
- Intravenous phentolamine appears predictive of success with subsequent sympathetic blocks but is rarely used these days.

Just as with adults the following drugs are sometimes used successfully for this condition, but very little is published regarding their use in children:

- Tricyclic antidepressants
- Anticonvulsants
- NMDA blockers, ketamine
- A trial of epidural clonidine may be useful in severe cases
- Local anaesthetics
- Adenosine is an endogenous substance with an inhibitory effect on the dorsal horn and may be useful for allodynia but less so for pain (Olsson 1999)
- Topical capsaicin. This substance may cause severe burning pain. High doses were effective in a study by Robbins et al. (1998), but this may be due to the regional anaesthesia under which it was given. Children rarely tolerate capsaicin
- Topical aspirin (Franklin & McRury 2003)

Non-pharmacological strategies
- Very careful and sensitive explanation to the child and his or her parents is needed. They may have experienced much frus-

tration and fear prior to a final diagnosis and many children and parents can feel that the problem has been dismissed as purely psychological.

- Physical therapy is vital to restore function as quickly as possible and reverse any dysfunction caused by inappropriate immobilisation that may have been occurring prior to diagnosis.
- This may need to be combined with a psychological programme based on cognitive behavioural therapy.
- TENS.
- Dorsal column stimulation.

Many of the other non-pharmacological strategies previously mentioned may also be helpful.

Resources

Help groups for children and parents, with lots of other useful website links for patients, clinicians and academics:

- Support Kids In Pain (SKIP): www.shsskip.swan.ac.uk/home (accessed September 2005)
- Medline Plus: www.nlm.nih.gov/medlineplus/reflexsympatheticdystrophy (accessed September 2005)
- National Institute of Neurological Disorders and Stroke: www.ninds. nih.gov/disorders/reflex_sympathetic_dystrophy/detail_reflex_sympathetic_ dystrophy (accessed September 2005)
- Complex regional pain syndrome: www.rsd-arena.co.uk/4520 (accessed September 2005). A useful site for patients

---

Chronic musculoskeletal or body wall pain

Sources of chronic musculoskeletal or body wall pain in children include:

- Juvenile rheumatoid arthritis. See Chapter 5 for treatment in older children.
- Fibromyalgia. See Chapter 6 for treatment in adults.

Pharmacological strategies

Following the basic principles for multimodal analgesia will establish whether a child's chronic pain will respond to analgesia. Strong opioids in children are best only used when all other strategies have failed and only if the child is showing demonstrable benefit in terms of improving function, mobility, mood, social interaction, etc. As with adults, opioids for chronic pain sufferers need to be managed by a knowledgeable and experienced clinician who can follow up the child on a regular basis to monitor progress.

Non-pharmacological strategies

As well as the strategies for adults and children covered previously or in subsequent chapters, there has been some literature published on the use of acupuncture and hypnosis for chronic pain which may offer some benefit to selected children. As with most complementary therapies, more research is needed to establish exactly which children may benefit most (Zelter et al. 2002).

Resources
- Eccleston et al. (2002) for information on psychosocial therapy
- Zelter et al. (2002) for information on acupuncture and hypnosis

Chronic visceral pain

For the majority of these children treatment will be centred on psychosocial factors, with emphasis on family reaction and behaviour and the development of effective coping strategies. For some this may require a specialist referral to a multidisciplinary team ideally including a psychologist skilled in the implementation and evaluation of these strategies.

- Chest pain – asthma, chronic bronchitis, allergic cough (see Chapter 5).
- Inflammatory bowel disease (see Chapter 5).
- Recurrent and chronic abdominal pain. This is common in children but in most cases a specific organic diagnosis cannot be found (Apley & Nalsh 1958). This apparent lack of organic pathology to explain symptoms has forced researchers to consider the influence of psychosocial factors. A population-based cohort study looked at the influence of anxious family members or the presence of other family members with physical ill health on chronic abdominal pain in children (Hotopf et al. 1998, p. 1196) and concluded the following:
  — Persistent abdominal pain in childhood is more common in families with high rates of reported physical illness and psychological symptoms.

— Children with persistent abdominal pain are not at increased risk of developing physical symptoms in adulthood.
— Abdominal pain in childhood is associated with increased risk of psychiatric disorders in adulthood such as anxiety and depression.

Resources

- Campo et al. (2004) for information on abdominal pain, anxiety and depression
- Garber et al. (1990) for information on abdominal pain, psychiatric diagnosis and parental psychopathology
- Plunkett & Beattie (2005) for information on abdominal pain
- Robinson et al. (1990) for information on the impact of life events, family history and abdominal pain
- Subcommittee on Chronic Abdominal Pain (2005)
- Walker & Greene (1989) and Walker et al. (1993) for further information on abdominal pain, the family, depression and anxiety

---

Sickle cell disease

Sickle cell disease affects children from certain ethnic groups and is responsible for significant pain. Box 4.4 details a research study that looked at the characteristics of pain associated with the disease.

The disease can manifest itself in many different ways; the more common sources of pain with this condition are listed below:

- Vaso-occlusive episodes causing ischaemic pain and cramping
- Bone infarction
- Bone marrow infarction
- Osteomyelitis
- Cholecystitis
- Acute chest syndrome

Box 4.4 Pain experienced by children with sickle cell disease

Data were collected from 60 children aged 3–60 months with sickle cell disease over a three year period. Each month parents/guardians were asked about their children's pain. Thirty seven of the 60 children experienced at least one episode of pain lasting from half a day to 19 days, with the average episode lasting 2 days or less. The abdomen and legs were the most common locations of pain. Parents or guardians gave medication and non-pharmacological strategies such as warm baths and massage. See Ely et al. (2005)

- Bowel infarction
- Inflicted pain associated with treatments such as biopsies or multiple venepuncture

Principles of assessment and evaluation for sickle cell disease

No specific tools appear to be particularly recommended for this condition, but a pain diary kept by the child or parents may be useful. It may give a running guide to help indicate whether a pain is caused by the patient's known condition or whether it is not typical. What analgesics have been tried so far and which ones have been successful can be documented. Other factors could include the impact of the pain in terms of distress and loss of schooling, etc. Most children like to use smiley faces, colours or even a traffic lights illustration to help indicate the severity of pain. Whatever the child is used to should be fine as numbers or faces are easily graded from no pain to severe pain. It helps children, health care providers and parents to record the information listed below in a daily diary where pain flares.

A tip is to remember the acronym **LOCATES** which has been developed to assist in pain assessment in children with a sickle cell crisis (Georgia Comprehensive Sickle Cell Center at Grady Health System 2005).

- **L – Location:** note the exact location of the pain and describe if it travels anywhere
- **O – Other Symptoms:** record any other symptoms such as fever, nausea, cough
- **C – Character:** describe the pain, e.g. deep, burning, throbbing
- **A – Aggravating and Alleviating Things:** what makes pain better or worse?
- **T – Timing:** when did pain start, has it been there all the time or does it fluctuate?
- **E – Environment and Effect:** location and activity when the pain started. How does it affect daily routine?
- **S – Severity:** rate how much pain on a 0 to 10 or similar scale

During a severe attack of pain patients must be treated as emergencies. In the past children and their families suffering from sickle cell disease have encountered unhelpful barriers to effective pain management. Because the condition is usually confined to patients of African decent, ethnocultural disparity between patient and health care provider has been blamed. In addition, unfounded concerns about opioid addiction and the potential for opioid diversion, i.e. opioids being obtained and then sold on to addicts, have influenced the use of the most effective drugs for managing this very painful condition. Unfortunately undertreatment of pain has lead to mistrust by patients and their families, often leading to manipulative and dramatic behaviour in order to try to obtain pain relief. Ideally patients require specialist knowledge in a health care centre familiar to them and their condition.

Pharmacological strategies
Mild to moderate pain may be treated with paracetamol or an NSAID such as ibuprofen. Severe pain may need a strong opioid either given orally or titrated intravenously until adequate analgesia is achieved or side effects limit further titration. Caution is needed with paracetamol if used long term or in high doses as it is hepatoxic and its effect on the liver if used chronically in these children is unknown. NSAIDs also pose problems, particularly the risk of gastric bleeding, which may be worse in children with sickle cell disease who have reduced levels of haemoglobin. The newer Cox-2 inhibitors may prove a viable alternative as they appear to have a better side effect profile for gastrointestinal bleeding, clotting disorders and renal problems. Recent evidence in cardiovascular disease means these drugs, not yet licensed for children, need more research.

Local anaesthetics should be used for all needle procedures as children will require frequent cannulation. EMLA cream requires an occlusive dressing and approximately 60 minutes to work. Amethocaine gel has a more rapid onset of action (Lawson et al. 1995). Morphine appears in most contemporary publications to be the gold standard, and if given via a PCA for severe acute flares of pain requiring hospitalisation, an indication of effective dosing levels is provided. Often this is much higher than that normally required by children postoperatively. Long-acting oral opioids and patches may gain popularity in the future once pain is controlled. The use of opioids such as pethidine or agonist-antagonists such as pentazocine is now questioned.

Non-pharmacological strategies

Patients and families have frequently used cognitive-behavioural and physical activities in addition to oral analgesics to treat sickle cell-related pain at home. However, a study by Dampier et al. (2004) concluded that patients and parents may benefit from additional training and support to make the most of non-pharmacological therapies. The use of psychological, social and behavioural components of treatment are also now finding their way into the treatment of sickle cell disease in British hospitals (Thomas 2000) and can aid in the treatment of chronic pain by reducing psychological distress and boosting confidence. Self-hypnosis may also have a place with these children (Dinges et al. 1997). Many Accident and Emergency Departments recognise the time delays in prescribing analgesics and have started using stickers to flag up the need for opioid prescriptions. This can help to allay fear and anxiety for patients and their families.

Resources

- Guidelines for managing a painful sickle cell crisis are available from the British Association for Accident and Emergency Medicine (BAEM) via the Pain Talk website: www.gb42.com/ynotsickle.html (accessed September 2005)
- Sickle cell disease information for school personnel: Special Child Health and Early Intervention Services, New Jersey Department of Health and Senior Services: www.state.nj.us/health/fhs/sicklecell (accessed September 2005)

The following may be useful for those wanting to know more about the condition itself:

- American Family Physician, *Sickle Cell Disease in Childhood. Part I. Laboratory Diagnosis, Pathophysiology and Health Maintenance*: www.aafp.org (accessed September 2005)
- American Family Physician, Sickle Cell Disease in Childhood. Part II. Diagnosis and Treatment of Major Complications and Recent Advances in Treatment: www.aafp.org (accessed September 2005)
- MedlinePlus: *Sickle Cell Anaemia*: www.nlm.nih.gov/medlineplus (accessed September 2005)
- American Pain Society (1999) *Guideline for the Management of Acute and Chronic Pain in Sickle Cell Disease*. American Pain Society, Glenview, Illinois
- Jacob (2001) and Stinson & Naser (2003) for information on pain management during crisis
- Thomas et al. (1998) for information on the role of cognitive behavioural therapy
- Zelter et al. (2002) for information on acupuncture and hypnosis

---

SUMMARY

Children and adolescents bring their own challenges for health care professionals trying to establish good pain management. Crucial to the implementation of any effective strategy is communication and finding ways of doing this effectively. Family and close friends will usually be helpful in assisting health care professionals select a useful pain assessment tool and will often participate in care. They may be the first to notice changes in behaviour and attitude that could be a sign of inadequate pain control. Research continues to support interventions, but many painful conditions have been neglected. The role of the nurse is central to ensuring effective communication and the selection and utilisation of a range of strategies.

REFERENCES

Apley, J. & Nalsh, N. (1958) Recurrent abdominal pains: a field study of 1000 school children. *Archives of Diseases in Childhood* **33**, 165–170.

Attard, A.R., Corlett, M.J., Kidner, N.J., Leslie, A.P. & Fraser, I.A. (1992) Safety of early pain relief for acute abdominal pain. *British Medical Journal* **305**, 554–556.

Baker, C. & Wong, D. (1987) QUEST: a process of pain assessment in children. *Orthopaedic Nurse* **6** (1), 11–21.

Beyer, J.E. & Aradine, C.R. (1986) Content validity of an instrument to measure young children's perceptions of their pain. *Paediatric Nurse* **1**, 386–395.

Bieri, D., Reeve, R.A., Champion, G.D., Addicoat, L. & Ziegler, J.B. (1990) The Faces Pain Scale for self-assessment of the severity of pain experienced by children: development, initial validation and preliminary investigation for ratio scale properties. *Pain* **41**, 139–150.

Borland, M.L., Jacobs, I. & Geelhoed, G. (2002) Intranasal fentanyl reduces acute pain in children in the emergency department: a safety and efficacy study. *Emergency Medicine* **14** (3), 275–280.

Brown, L., Denmark, T.K., Wittlake, W.A., Vargas, E.J., Watson, T. & Crabb, J.W. (2004) Procedural sedation use in the ED: management of paediatric ear and nose foreign bodies. American Journal of *Emergency Medicine* **22** (4), 310–314.

Campo, C.V., Bridge, J., Ehmann, M., et al. (2004) Recurrent abdominal pain, anxiety, and depression in primary care. *Pediatrics* **113** (4), 817–824.

Dampier, C., Ely, E., Eggleston, B., Brodecki, D. & O'Neal, P. (2004) Physical and cognitive-behavioral activities used in the home management of sickle pain: a daily diary study in children and adolescents. *Pediatric Blood Cancer* **43** (6), 674–678.

Dangel, T. (2005) Management of chronic pain in children. *Current Paediatrics* **15** (1), 69–74.

Davies, M. & Crawford, I. (2001) Nasal diamorphine for acute pain relief in children. *British Medical Journal* **18**, 27.

Dinges, D.F., Whitehouse, W.G., Orne, E.C., et al. (1997) Self-hypnosis training as an adjunctive treatment in the management of pain associated with sickle cell disease. *International Journal of Clinical and Experimental Hypnosis* **45** (4), 417–432.

Eccleston, C., Morley, S., Williams, A., Yorke, L. & Mastroyannopoulou, K. (2002) Systematic review of randomised controlled trials of psychological therapy for chronic pain in children and adolescents, with a subset meta-analysis of pain relief. *Pain* **99**, 1–2, 157–165.

Eland, J. (1985) The child who is hurting. *Seminars in Oncology Nursing* **1**, 116–122.

Ely, B., Dampier, C., Brodecki, D., O'Neal, P. & Coleman, C. (2005) Characteristics of pain episodes in infants and young children with sickle cell disease. *Journal of Pain* **6** (3, Suppl. 1).

Finley, G.A. & McGrath, P.J. (1997) *The Measurement of Pain in Infants and Children. Progress in Pain Research and Management*, vol. 10. IASP Press, Seattle.

Franck, L. & Jones, M. (2003) Computer-taught coping techniques for venepuncture: preliminary findings from usability testing with children, parents and staff. *Journal of Child Health Care* **7** (1), 41–54.

Franklin, G.F. & McRury, S. (2003) P434 topical aspirin for the treatment of neuropathic pain. *European Journal of Internal Medicine* **14** (1), S154.

Garber, J., Zeman, J. & Walker, L.S. (1990) Recurrent abdominal pain in children: psychiatric diagnoses and parental psychopathology. *Journal of the American Academy of Child and Adolescent Psychiatry* **29**, 648–656.

Georgia Comprehensive Sickle Cell Center at Grady Health System (2005) *The Pneumonic LOCATES is Used to Assist in Pain Assessment in Children with a Sickle Cell Crisis. From Pain Assessment and Pain Management in Sickle Cell*. Available at www.scinfo.org, accessed September 2005.

Gold, J., Reger, G., Rizzo, A., Buckwalter, G., Kim, S. & Joseph, M. (2005) *Virtual reality in outpatient phlebotomy: evaluating paediatric pain distraction during blood draw*. In: Proceedings of American Pain Society Conference, Boston, 30 March–2 April.

Goodman, J.E. & McGrath, P.J. (1991) The epidemiology of pain in children and adolescents: a review. *Pain* **46**, 247–264.

Graumuller, S. & Laudien, B. (2003) Postoperative pain after tonsillectomy – comparison of children and adults. *International Congress Series* **1254**, 469–472.

Harreby, M., Neegaard, K., Hesselsce, G. & Kjer, J. (1995) Are radiological changes in thoracic and lumbar spine of adolescents risk factors for low back pain in adults? *Spine* **20**, 2298–2302.

Hester, N.O. (1979) The preoperative child's reaction to immunization. *Nursing Research* **28**, 250–255.

Hester, N.O., Foster, R. & Kristensen, K. (1990) Measurement of pain in children; generalizability and validity of the pain ladder and the poker chip tool. In: Tyler, D.C. & Krane, E.J. (eds) *Advances in Pain Research and Therapy*, 79–84. Raven Press, New York.

Hoffman, H.G., Patterson, J.N., Carrougher, D.R. & Furness, G.T. III (2000) Virtual reality as an adjunctive pain control during burn wound care in adolescent patients. *Pain* **85** (1), 305–309.

Hoffman, H.G., Sharar, S.R., Coda, B., et al. (2004) Manipulating presence influences the magnitude of virtual reality analgesia. *Pain* **111** (1–2), 162–168.

Hotopf, M., Carr, S., Mayou, R., Wadsworth, M. & Wessely, S. (1998) Why do children have chronic abdominal pain, and what happens to them when they grow up? Population based cohort study. *British Medical Journal* **316** (18), 1196–1200.

Huth, M.M., Broome, M.E. & Good, M. (2004) Imagery reduces children's post-operative pain. *Pain* **110** (1–2), 439–448.

Jacob, E. (2001) Pain management in sickle cell disease. *Pain Management Nursing* **2** (4), 121–131.

Jay, S.M., Elliot, C.H., Ozolina, M., Olson, R.A. & Pruitt, S.D. (1985) Behavioural management of children's distress during painful medical procedures. *Behaviour Research and Therapy* **23** (1), 513–520.

Jylli, L., Lundeberg, S. & Olsson, G.L. (2002) Retrospective evaluation of continuous epidural infusion for postoperative pain in children. *Acta Anaesthesiologica Scandinavica* **46** (6), 654–659.

Kaygusuz, I. & Susaman, N. (2003) The effects of dexamethasone, bupivacaine and topical lidocaine spray on pain after tonsillectomy. *International Journal of Pediatric Otorhinolaryngology* **67** (7), 737–742.

Kim, C.S. (2002) *Postgraduate Medicine On Line: Musculoskeletal Pain in Adolescents. Diagnostic Criteria are Distinct from those in Adults.* Available at www.postgradmed.com/issues/2002/04_02/kim (accessed September 2005).

Kim, S., Gold, J., Rizzo, A. & Kant, A. (2005) *Effectiveness of virtual reality for paediatric pain distraction during i.v. placement.* In: Proceedings of American Pain Society Conference, Boston. 30 March–2 April.

Lawson, R.A., Smart, N.G., Gudgeon, A.C. & Morton, N.S. (1995) Evaluation of an amethocaine gel preparation for percutaneous analgesia before venous cannulation in children. *British Journal of Anaesthesia* **75**, 282–285.

McGrath, P.J. & Finley, G.A. (eds) (1999) *Chronic and Recurrent Pain in Children and Adolescents.* IASP Press, Seattle.

McKenzie, I.M., Gaukroger, P.B., Ragg, P.G. & Brown, T.C.K. (eds) (1997) *Manual of Acute Pain Management in Children.* Churchill Livingstone, New York.

Meh, D. & Denislic, M. (1998) Subclinical neuropathy in type 1 diabetic children. *Electroencephalography and Clinical Neurophysiology*, **109**, 274–280.

Mitchell, P. (1985) Critically ill children: the importance of touch in a high technological environment. *Nursing Admininstration Quarterly* **9** (4), 38–46.

Moir, M.S., Bair, E., Shinnick, P. & Messner, A. (2000) Acetaminophen versus acetaminophen with codeine after pediatric tonsillectomy. *Laryngoscope* **110**, 1824–1827.

Morton, N.S. (1998) *Acute Paediatric Pain Management. A Practical Guide*. W.B. Saunders, London.

Murphy, S., Buckle, P. & Stubbs, D. (2004) Classroom posture and self-reported back and neck pain in schoolchildren. *Applied Ergonomics* **35** (2), 113–120.

Olsen, D., Andrews, R.L., Dearwater, S.R., et al. (1992) The epidemiology of low back pain in an adolescent population. *American Journal of Public Health* **82** (4), 606–608.

Olsson, G.L. (1999) Neuropathic pain in children. In: McGrath, P.J. & Finley, G.A. (eds) (1999) *Chronic and Recurrent Pain in Children and Adolescents*. IASP Press, Seattle, pp. 75–98.

Olsson, G.L. & Berde, C.B. (1993) Neuropathic pain in children and adolescents. In: Schecter, N.K., Berde, C.B. & Yaster, M. (eds) *Pain in Infants, Children and Adolescents*. Williams and Wilkins, Baltimore, pp. 473–493.

Pace, S. & Burke, T.F. (1996) Intravenous morphine for early pain relief in patients with acute abdominal pain. *Academic Emergency Medicine* **3**, 1086–1092.

Palermo, T.M., Valenzuela, D. & Stork, P. (2004a) A randomized trial of electronic versus paper pain diaries in children: impact on compliance, accuracy, and acceptability. *Pain* **107** (3), 213–219.

Palermo, T.M., Witherspoon, D., Valenzuela, D. & Drotar, D.D. (2004b) Development and validation of the Child Activity Limitations Interview: a measure of pain-related functional impairment in school-age children and adolescents. *Pain* **109** (3), 461–470.

Peden, V., Choonara, E. & Vater, M. (2005) Validating the Derbyshire Children's Hospital Pain Tool in children aged 6–12 years. *Journal of Child Health Care* **1** (9), 59–71.

Peters, J.W., Bandell Hoekstra, I.E., Huijer Abu-Saad, H., Bouwmeester, J., Meursing, A.E. & Tibboel, D. (1999) Patient controlled analgesia in children and adolescents: a randomized controlled trial. *Paediatric Anesthesia* **9** (3), 235–241.

Plunkett, A. & Beattie, R.M. (2005) Recurrent abdominal pain in childhood. *Journal of the Royal Society of Medicine* **98** (3), 1, 101–106.

Pölkki, T., Vehviläinen-Julkunen, K. & Pietilä, A.M. (2001) Non-pharmacological methods in relieving children's postoperative pain: a survey on hospital nurses in Finland. *Journal of Advanced Nursing* **34** (4), 483–492.

Pölkki, T., Pietila, A.M. & Vehvilainnen-Julkunen, K. (2003) Hospitalized children's descriptions of their experiences with post surgical pain relieving methods. *International Journal of Nursing Studies* **40** (1), 33–44.

Qureshi, J. & Buckingham, S. (1994) A pain assessment tool for all children. *Paediatric Nurse* **6** (7), 11–13.

Robbins, W.R., Staats, P.S., Levine, J., et al. (1998) Treatment of intractable pain with topical large-dose capsaicin, preliminary report. *Anesthesia and Analgesia* **86**, 579–583.

Robinson, J.O., Alvarez, J.H. & Dodge, J.A. (1990) Life events and family history in children with recurrent abdominal pain. *Journal of Psychosomatic Research* **34**, 171–181.

Romsing, J., Hertel, S., Harder, A. & Rasmussen, M. (1998) Examination of acetaminophen for outpatient management of postoperative pain in children. *Pediatric Anesthesia* **8** (3), 235–239.

Romsing, J., Ostergaard, D., Drozdziewicz, D., Schultz, P. & Ravn, G. (2000) Diclofenac or acetaminophen for analgesia in paediatric tonsillectomy outpatients. *Acta Anaesthesiologica Scandinavica* **44** (3), 291–295.

Royal College of Paediatrics and Child Health (1999) *Medicines for Children*. RCPCH, London.

Salminen, J.J., Pentti, J. & Terho, P. (1992) Low back pain and disability in 14 year old schoolchildren. *Acta Paediatrica* 81, 1035–1039.

Savedra, M.C., Holzemer, W.L., Tesler, M.D. & Wilkie, D.J. (1993) Assessment of post operative pain in children and adolescents using the adolescent paediatric pain tool. *Nursing Research* **42** (1), 5–9.

Schmidt, A., Bjorkman, S. & Akeson, J. (2001) Preoperative rectal diclofenac versus paracetamol for tonsillectomy: effects on pain and blood loss. *Acta Anaesthesiologica Scandinavica* **45** (1), 48–52.

Scholer, S.J., Pituch, K., Orr, D.P. & Dittus, R.S. (1999) Test ordering on children with acute abdominal pain. *Clinical Pediatrics* **38**, 493–497.

Somdas, M.A., Senturk, M., Ketenci, I., Erkorkmaz, U. & Unlu, Y. (2004) Efficacy of bupivacaine for post-tonsillectomy pain: a study with the intra-individual design. *International Journal of Pediatric Otorhinolaryngology* **68** (11), 1391–1395.

Stella, J., Ellis, R. & Sprivulis, P. (2000) Nerve stimulator-assisted femoral nerve block in the emergency department. *Emergency Medicine* **12** (4), 322–325.

Stinson, J. & Naser, B. (2003) Pain management in children with sickle cell disease. *Paediatric Drugs* **5** (4), 229–241.

Subcommittee on Chronic Abdominal Pain (2005) Chronic abdominal pain in children. *Pediatrics* **115** (3), e370–e381.

Sutters, K.A., Miaskowski, C., Holdridge-Zeuner, D., et al. (2004) A randomized clinical trial of the effectiveness of a scheduled oral analgesic dosing regimen for the management of postoperative pain in children following tonsillectomy. *Pain* **110** (1–2), 49–55.

Thomas, V. (2000) Cognitive behavioural therapy in pain management for sickle cell disease. *International Journal of Palliative Nursing* **6** (9), 434–442.

Thomas, V.N., Wilson-Barnett, J. & Goodhart, F.J. (1998) The role of cognitive-behavioural therapy in the management of pain in patients with sickle cell disease. *Journal of Advanced Nursing* **27** (5),1002–1009.

Twycross, A. (1998) The management of acute pain in children. *Professional Nurse* **14** (2), 95–98.

Twycross, A., Moriarty, A. & Betts, T. (eds) (1997) Paediatric Pain Management. A Multi-disciplinary Approach. Radcliffe Medical Press, Oxford.

Varni, J.W., Thompson, K.L. & Hanson, V. (1987) The Varni-Thompson Paediatric Pain Questionnaire 1: chronic musculoskeletal pain in juvenile rheumatoid arthritis. *Pain* **28**, 27–38.

Varni, J.W., Waldron, S.A., Gragg, R.A., et al. (1996) Development of the Waldron/Varni Pediatric Pain Coping Inventory. Pain, **67** (1), 141–150.

Walker, L.S. & Greene, J.W. (1989) Children with recurrent abdominal pain and their parents: more somatic complaints, anxiety, and depression than other patient families? *Journal of Pediatric Psychology* **14**, 231–243.

Walker, L.S., Garber, J. & Greene, J.W. (1993) Psychosocial correlates of recurrent childhood pain: a comparison of pediatric patients with recurrent abdominal pain, organic illness and psychiatric disorders. *Journal of Abnormal Psychology* **102**, 248–258.

Walker, L.S., Garber, J., Van Slyke, D.A. & Greene, J.W. (1995) Long-term health outcomes in patients with recurrent abdominal pain. *Journal of Pediatric Psychology* **20**, 233–245.

Walker, S. & Eyres, R. (1997) Acute management of complex regional pain syndrome type 1. In: McKenzie, I., Gaukroger, P.B., Ragg, P. & Brown, T.C.K. (Kester) (eds) *Manual of Acute Pain Management in Children*. Churchill Livingstone, New York.

Wilder, R.T., Berde, C.B., Wolohan, M., Vieyra, M.A., Masek, B.J. & Micheli, L.J. (1992) Reflex sympathetic dystrophy in children. *Journal of Bone and Joint Surgery* **6**, 910–919.

Wilson, J.A., Kendall, J.M. & Cornelius, P. (1997) Intranasal diamorphine for paediatric analgesia: assessment of safety and efficacy. *Journal of Accident and Emergency Medicine* **14** (2), 70–72.

Zeltzer, L.K. & LeBaron, D.S. (1982) Hypnosis and nonhypnotic techniques for reduction of pain and anxiety during painful procedures in children and adolescents with cancer. *Journal of Pediatrics* **101**, 1032–1035.

Zeltzer, L.K., Tsao, J.C.I., Stelling, C., Powers, M., Levy, S. & Waterhouse, M. (2002) A phase I study on the feasibility and acceptability of an acupuncture/hypnosis intervention for chronic pediatric pain. *Journal of Pain and Symptom Management* **24** (4), 437–446.

Zoltie, N. & Cust, M.P. (1986) Analgesia in the acute abdomen. *Annals of the Royal College of Surgeons of England* **68**, 209–210.

Pain in Early Adulthood (12–18 Years)   **5**

INTRODUCTION

This chapter discusses pain problems experienced most often by young people, as they grow through late childhood into early adulthood (12–18 years). Their needs both physically, psychologically and socially are complex at this time and the effective management of pain requires skilled sensitivity and sound knowledge. Acute pain is frequently experienced through sports injuries, erupting wisdom teeth, menstruation (for girls) and 'growing pains'. The years of adolescence and early adulthood are not usually associated with chronic or particularly challenging pain, but arthritis and sickle cell disease can be as prevalent within this age group as it is in younger children. Historically, the management of pain in young people has been inadequate and although improvements have been made, research continues to highlight problems (see Box 5.1).

Box 5.1 Prevalence of acute pain in Sweden

In Sweden, a country with an excellent reputation for the quality of their health care, a nationwide survey revealed that 17% of children had moderate or severe pain following surgery. A further 31% of children reported moderate or severe acute pain not associated with surgery. Organisational problems and poor education of doctors and nurses were the major causes identified. See Karling et al. (2002).

LEARNING OBJECTIVES

❏ To understand some of the physiological and psychosocial factors that impact on the perception and management of pain in young adults

❏ To identify some of the changes in puberty that may make adolescents more vulnerable to pain

❏ To recognise the special needs that apply in order to improve communication and pain assessment in this age group

❏ To explore several common painful conditions and the interventions that may be appropriate for the young adult

ACUTE PAIN

Physiological changes

Commonly, acute pain in this age group is associated with trauma due to sprains and strains experienced during sports and leisure activity. Some children will battle with the inevitable acute flares of pain associated with chronic conditions such as sickle cell disease or juvenile arthritis.

Principles of assessment and evaluation for acute pain

Children's perceptions of pain are influenced by their developmental age, culture, personality and their previous experiences, etc. A valid and appropriate pain assessment tool negotiated with the teenager is probably going to be the most effective. They may not always be forthcoming about their pain and may want to appear tough and resilient. Alternatively they may be very demanding with totally unrealistic expectations of what may be achievable. Selection of a pain assessment tool should always incorporate a pain scale. Most children over 12 years old will prefer a similar tool to that used by adults, but they should be encouraged to choose one from the following examples that they feel most comfortable with:

- Visual analogue scale (VAS)
- Verbal graphic rating scale
- Numerical rating scale
- Pain thermometer
- Faces scale (more usually preferred by younger children)
- The Word-graphic rating scale (evaluated for children and adolescents' pain) (Tesler et al. 1997)
- Adolescent Paediatric Pain Tool (APPT) (Savedra et al. 1999)

The Royal College of Nurses provides clinical practice guidelines on the recognition and assessment of acute pain in children (RCN 2003), while Gillies et al. (1997, 1999) provides information on assessment and management of pain in adolescents.

Surgery

There is good evidence that acute postoperative pain for adolescents remains inadequately managed in hospitals (Gillies et al. 1999), despite it being relatively easy to control in young people who are unlikely to be chronically ill or have their treatment strategies complicated by the need for polypharmacy. Older children and young adults may start to take some responsibility for their own pain management but may lack the confidence to follow advice or instructions from health care professionals. There is also good evidence that when parents take this responsibility, they fail to provide adequate analgesia for their children even when they have received specific instructions on post-surgical pain management (Finley et al. 1996; Chambers et al. 1997).

Unfortunately adolescents may also be particularly affected by the lack of formal training in adolescent health care and a poor understanding of their analgesic needs by health care professionals. The study by Gillies et al. (1999) particularly highlights common misconceptions held by health care professionals toward adolescents. For example, the request for pain relief was seen as attention-seeking. Not only did nurses underestimate analgesic requirements, but also, by mistaken beliefs or negative attitudes, they suggested a request for pain relief was 'clock-watching for drugs'. 'Postoperative pain is not all that sore. (It's) not in the same league as labour or renal colic' one nurse is quoted as saying (Gillies et al. 1999, p. 213). Attitudes such as this impede effective pain management.

Examples of common procedures performed on young adults

- Hernia repair
- Appendicectomy
- Tonsillectomy

- Adenoidectomy
- Trauma surgery to repair bones or soft tissues
- Laparotomy
- Plastic surgery following burns
- Dental surgery to remove large molars and wisdom teeth
- Abscess drainage

Experiencing postoperative pain (short stay)

Case study

James aged 14 has been admitted to the Day Case Unit for removal of metal work from his previously fractured femur under a general anaesthetic. He is very fearful as his initial surgery proved very painful postoperatively. Everything goes well, but on waking his pain score remains high despite being given 5 mg of morphine intraoperatively and a full dose of paracetamol and ibuprofen in the recovery room. The nurses have a preprescribed drug chart that enables them to administer additional IV morphine on a milligram per kilogram basis and they are able to establish effective pain control but only at the maximum dose prescribed. James is closely monitored in recovery. His respiratory rate and sedation remain perfectly stable and he is returned to the ward after 40 minutes. He makes a full, event-free and relatively comfortable recovery but continues to require regular full doses of analgesia for 7 days.

As we know from work with neonates and small children, previous experiences of pain may leave an imprint on the central nervous system, making it hypersensitive to subsequent painful experiences. Treating James' pain more aggressively using multimodal analgesia as soon as it was reported in the recovery room may well have contributed to his more effective pain control in the postoperative period. It is not unusual for patients to report pain for at least 7 days after what health care professionals may regard as routine and relatively minor surgery (Romsing et al. 2000).

Experiencing postoperative pain (longer stay)

Case study

Clare aged 15 returns to the ward following a laparotomy to remove her spleen after a road traffic accident. She has a thoracic epidural in situ with a solution of bupivacaine and fentanyl running at a rate of 8 ml per hour. She is comfortable at rest but has some pain on movement. Her blood pressure has been a little low so rather than increase the epidural rate at this stage she is given one IV dose of paracetamol. When she is able to tolerate oral fluids a few hours later, she is also prescribed regular paracetamol orally and this multimodal strategy optimises her pain control.

Pharmacological strategies

An epidural combining a local anaesthetic with an opioid will usually provide the most effective analgesia following a laparotomy that requires a midline incision. PCA alone or even with a background infusion does not appear to offer effective analgesia when used for more major surgery in children and adolescents (Peters et al. 1999). PCA may be useful if an epidural has to be discontinued or fails within 24–48 hours postoperatively or before oral analgesia can be tolerated.

Paracetamol is always a good basic analgesic with a loading dose of either oral 20 mg/kg prior to surgery or rectal 30 g/kg following induction of analgesia, then reverting to 10–15 mg/kg. The introduction of IV paracetamol to the UK in 2004 has enabled many patients unable to tolerate oral or rectal analgesia to benefit from this useful drug. The addition of paracetamol contributes to balanced analgesia, possibly reducing the need for a high volume epidural and reducing the risk of side effects such as hypotension and loss of sensation.

Once the epidural is discontinued, consider the use of stickers for children with acute pain to ensure that a full therapeutic dose of a range of analgesics on a milligram per kilogram (mg per kg) basis is given regularly until pain subsides (see Fig. 4.3).

Box 5.2 Comparing postoperative pain experiences

Trip et al. (2003) compared the pain and coping strategies after surgery of 10 adolescents and 10 adults. Their study found significant differences in pain, catastrophising and coping between the two groups. Catastrophising was a strong factor in the differences in pain (adolescents experiencing more pain and catastrophising). They suggest that preferred coping styles, such as wanting information before and after surgery or avoiding information about the procedure and using distraction afterwards, should be identified and pain interventions tailored to match the adolescent's needs.

Non-pharmacological strategies

Older children usually thrive if kept mentally occupied as much as possible. Access to computers, 'gameboys', television, videos, CDs and a radio can be very helpful. Visits from friends and family can also help to reduce the perceived intensity and unpleasantness of pain. Teenagers usually benefit from feeling they have some control and need to be kept informed of what has happened and what to expect (see Box 5.2). These distractions do not replace the need for regular analgesics but may help to enhance their effect.

Trauma

- Fractures
- Lacerations
- Foreign bodies
- Burns and scalds
- Road traffic accidents

Experiencing acute trauma pain

Case study

Barry aged 16 is admitted to hospital following an accident whilst riding his bicycle. He was coming down a hill and was in collision with a bus. He was not wearing a helmet. He has lacerations, multiple fractures and head and facial injuries and has been transferred to the High Dependency Unit. He is conscious, self-ventilating and stable. He is expected to make a full recovery but will need plastic surgery at a later date for his disfiguring facial injuries.

Teenagers who experience a traumatic injury can be left feeling very frightened. The strong emotions they feel during adolescence result in them handling trauma quite differently. Younger children depend directly on their family, whereas teenagers look more to their peer group for support. This can make their care and pain management more challenging. In Barry's case his pain will be potentially severe and protracted, possibly associated with significant distress about his future and body image. The following are examples of some of the issues that can contribute to the challenging nature of establishing effective analgesia in teenagers following a major trauma:

- Strong emotions such as sadness, anger, anxiety and guilt
- Exaggerated emotional reactions to small problems
- Constantly thinking about the traumatic event, with a need to talk about it often
- Sleep problems, including insomnia or sleeping more than usual
- Withdrawing from family and friends
- Wanting to spend more time alone
- Needing to be close to the family
- Increased need for independence
- Inability to cope with responsibilities or duties, reverting to immature or irresponsible behaviour
- Self-absorption, caring only about what is immediately important to them
- Loss of interest in life, school, friends and hobbies; they may become bored and listless
- Pessimistic outlook on life, unable to set goals
- Depression
- Cognitive changes, such as difficulties with short-term memory and concentration
- Restlessness, needing to be doing something or be with their peers all the time
- Angry, controlling, assertive and demanding
- Exaggeration of previous problems

Experiencing any severe trauma is going to be a challenge, but for teenagers it may be particularly difficult. They may rapidly change from being confident and independent to feeling insecure. This is confusing to teenagers themselves as well as parents and carers and will sometimes make communicating difficult. Teenagers may also not wish to share their fears, concerns and feelings with their parents as they may not wish to acknowledge the accident. This can upset their parents who may also need support during this difficult time. Providing effective analgesia relies on good communication skills and sensitivity to ensure that pain control is maintained. Teenagers appear to be able to communicate most effectively with their peers and this may help health care professionals to develop a strategy that includes close friends to assist in pain assessment. Teenagers will need plenty of reassurance that these reactions will subside in time and that you will work with them to ensure their recovery as quickly as possible:

- Give them accurate information about the accident and how their pain will be managed now and in the future. Keep them informed about how their recovery is progressing and how their pain will diminish as tissue heals.
- Encourage them to express their emotions and feelings and not suppress them.
- Keep communicating, explain about stress, recovery and how effective plastic and reconstructive surgery can be. It is ideal if there is somebody who can talk to them who has been through a similar experience. Reassure them about their future and that their current feelings and distress will pass.
- Do not get into arguments if they do not like how you are caring for them; instead ask them how else you can help.
- However hard, try to get them involved in something they enjoy and that can make them laugh.
- Maintain a routine that is secure and predictable. Try to keep changes to a minimum.

Sometimes teenagers have a narrower point of view than adults and can surprise us with their acceptance of trauma and injury. It may appear evident that the parents are experiencing greater suffering than the child, but they must be encouraged to try to not burden their child with their distress.

Pharmacological strategies

Following a head injury or following cranial surgery, codeine has been the traditional analgesic, although evidence for this drug in this situation is sparse. Caution with all opioids and sedative drugs has always been recommended as these drugs may confuse monitoring for sedation, conscious level and pupillary changes. Hypoxaemia and CO_2 mediated vascular intracranial pressure rises may be exacerbated by the narcotic CO_2 response. However, where other injuries occur, particularly to bone and soft tissue, rapid analgesia with strong IV opioids may be unavoidable as uncontrolled pain and the stress this can cause is also detrimental to recovery. Monitoring will have to be extremely vigilant to register any physiological changes.

A review by Roberts (2004) succinctly describes the dilemmas faced when trying to provide adequate analgesia with the most commonly used opioids of codeine, tramadol or morphine. Codeine is an unpredictable pro-drug (meaning a drug that is given in an inactive or significantly less active form and is metabolised in the body to its active form) and does not equate to a safe and effective analgesic post-craniotomy. There is a lack of evidence supporting tramadol and there are concerns over its interactions and side effects. The literature supports the use of morphine as an effective analgesic. When used in an environment that can ensure skilled monitoring, morphine should not be withheld, based on current evidence.

Children who have undergone significant trauma such as a major road traffic accident may be at risk of developing post-traumatic stress disorder with all the psychosocial implications this entails. One double blind, randomised study has evaluated the use of imipramine for children following burn injuries. These children developed post-traumatic stress disorder at a significantly lower rate than children who received chloral hydrate, a sedative (Robert et al. 1999). Saxe et al. (2001) undertook a study of child burn victims and demonstrated a significant relationship between the dosage of morphine received and a 6-month reduction in post-traumatic stress disorder symptoms. Whether these findings can be applied to other children who have been disfigured and face painful plastic surgery is unclear, but the possibility of depression and anxiety developing after a severe injury must always be considered.

Non-pharmacological strategies

In addition to the strategies outlined in the first part of this section, teenagers thrive on being kept occupied with the things they enjoy, such as films, music, magazines and their friends. Severely traumatised adolescents may also benefit from psychosocial interventions such as cognitive-behavioural therapy used as part of multimodal therapy (Foa et al. 1999). We are only just beginning to understand the negative impact that trauma may have, with MRI studies showing neurobiological alterations in the brains of adolescents exposed to significant stress (Yang et al. 2004).

Resources

- The Better Health Channel (2005), The Victorian (Australia) Government: www. betterhealth.vic.gov.au/bhcv2/bhcarticles.nsf/pages/trauma_and_teenagers_ common_reactions?opendocument (accessed October 2005)
- NICE Guideline, *Head Injury: Triage, Assessment, Investigation and Early Management of Head Injury in Infants, Children and Adults*: www.nice.org.uk/ pdf/cg4niceguideline.pdf (accessed October 2005). Unfortunately this guideline does not include pain relief although it is otherwise comprehensive
- Cohen (2003) for information on acute post-traumatic reactions
- Roberts (2004) for information on the safety of opioids post-craniotomy

---

Musculoskeletal or body wall pain

- Sprains
- Strains
- Compartment syndrome, where a muscle becomes too big for the muscle sheath, causing pain and possibly serious tissue damage. It may result from a blow or from a muscle tear that leads to bleeding and swelling into the muscle

Ligament injuries

These are usually treated with rest, ice, compression, elevation (RICE) and physical therapy. Most injuries to soft tissue will respond well to anti-inflammatory analgesics such as ibuprofen.

The following form the basic principles of managing ligament injury pain:

- Assess the cause, circumstances and extent of injury.
- Refer if necessary for emergency or specialised treatment.
- Initiate short-term treatment with **RICE (rest, ice, compression, elevation)**.
- Treat pain early with analgesics before it becomes established and administer regularly until pain subsides.
- Encourage early mobilisation, typically starting after 2 days' rest.
- Advise on prognosis and be positive. Recovery to usual function depends on the site and severity of the injury, as well as on levels of activity. For example, following a severe ankle sprain it can take a few weeks to be able to walk normally to school or college, but several months before an adolescent should be fully participating in sports activity.

Painful breast conditions

These are common during puberty and adolescence. In females, some breast changes or conditions are related to the menstrual cycle, while others may occur at any time. In this age group they are nearly always benign but may need further investigation and can cause distress and discomfort.

Cyclical breast pain

This is associated with the menstrual cycle and is nearly always hormonal. Hormones may not provide the total answer to cyclical breast pain, since it is often more severe in one breast than in the other. Encourage the adolescent to pre-empt the problem by keeping a diary. If the pain is cyclical, take simple analgesia early and regularly for a brief period of time. Sometimes they may need to use a trial and error approach to find a preparation that is most effective and suits them best. Non-steroidal anti-inflammatory drugs (NSAIDs) usually provide adequate analgesia if taken early. Topical NSAIDs may also be effective (Colak et al. 2003) and do not have the side effects of oral NSAIDs. Non-pharmacological strategies may also be important such as a good supportive bra and maintaining ideal weight. Although there is little scientific evidence, the following may also be useful in some breast pain sufferers: a diet rich in fruits, vegetables and grains, vitamins B_6, B_1 and E and evening primrose oil.

Cysts
Cysts often enlarge and become tender and painful just before the menstrual period. They are the most common reason for breast lumps in adolescents. They may be caused by a blockage in the breast glands and require draining. Plenty of reassurance may be necessary, but this may negate the need for regular pain control. Wearing a good supporting bra may be helpful, particularly for sport.

Fibroadenomas
Fibroadenomas are solid, smooth, firm, benign lumps that are most commonly found in women in their late teens and early twenties. Simple pain control with paracetamol may be all that is required if pain is troublesome.

Generalised breast lumps
These are sometimes termed 'fibrocystic disease' and 'fibroid breasts'. Many believe they are just part of the breast changes that many women undergo throughout the various stages of their lives and reassurance may well be all that is required.

Breast conditions in boys
Gynecomastia is a condition of painful breast enlargement in up to 50% of teenage boys and usually resolves after about 2 years once the adolescent growth spurt stops. Again, plenty of reassurance and simple analgesia as required are usually sufficient methods of managing pain.

Resources

- Prodigy: www.prodigy.nhs.uk/guidance.asp?gt=sprains%20and%20strains (accessed October 2005)
- Children's Hospital Boston, Massachusetts, Child Health, Breast Conditions: http://.web1.tch.harvard.edu/cfapps/a2ztopicdisplay.cfm?topic=breast%20 conditions (accessed October 2005)

Visceral pain

The following acute visceral pains in adolescents may require immediate treatment to rectify the condition. In addition the use of strong opioids may be required for severe pain in the more serious conditions where pain is failing to respond to non-opioids and adjuvant therapy.

Dysmenorrhoea

This is very common in girls and young women, associated with cramps or pain in the abdomen or back and possibly nausea, vomiting, diarrhoea, constipation, a headache or light-headedness. It is usually easy to treat with paracetamol, aspirin or ibuprofen. NSAIDs usually provide the most superior analgesia for this condition, which is related to prostaglandin production. However, which particular NSAID is most effective for the individual may require a trial-and-error approach, including in some cases a trial of a prescription-only NSAID or a Cox-2 if ibuprofen or aspirin are ineffective. When dysmenorrhoea is experienced every month on a regular basis then taking an NSAID 1–3 days prior to the onset of menstruation may be beneficial. For very severe pain, hormonal alteration of menstruation with oral contraceptives may offer a solution. Simple strategies should not be forgotten: exercise is thought to reduce cramping pain, a warm bath or a hot water bottle can also aid comfort and a diet high in omega three fatty acids is also thought to be helpful.

Threatened abortion

This may involve pain experienced in one or both lower quadrants. Pain may radiate to the lower back, buttocks, genitalia, perineum and suprapubic area. Paracetamol remains the safest drug to use in a viable pregnancy; however, its repeated use in later pregnancy has been linked to wheezing in early childhood (Shaheen et al. 2002). It is not known how relevant this is to the first trimester but its brief use does appear to be safe.

Ectopic pregnancy

This is not a viable pregnancy as the embryo is developing in the fallopian tube. The condition is life threatening and can cause extreme pain. Adolescents in particular may not know they are pregnant and be very frightened especially if the pregnancy rup-tures. Adequate pain control may well include a titrated strong IV opioid such as morphine to initiate pain control in addition to non-opioid analgesia until surgery can be performed.

Pelvic inflammatory disease
Initially, administering paracetamol regularly may be sufficient. If severe pain develops it can warrant additional analgesia. Anti-inflammatory treatment with corticoids such as dexamethasone (three tablets of 0.5 mg a day) or niflumic acid (Nifluril) (one 700 mg suppository per 12 hours) or NSAIDs such as or indomethacin (Indocid) (one 100 mg suppository twice a day) are suggested by Quentin & Lansac (2000). This should commence once the effectiveness of antibiotic therapy has been assessed from clinical signs. For severe pain, it would be inhumane to withhold analgesia until treatment begins to reduce the symp-toms and a trial of ibuprofen with its less adverse side effect profile may well be just as effective as indomethacin. Adolescents may also gain benefit from counselling regarding future sexual activity and fertility.

Chest pain
When teenagers complain of chest pain, most assume they have serious disease or cancer and are therefore very fearful. They usually report chest pain coming and going for several months, describing it as a sharp stab beneath the breastbone, and occur-ring with or without physical activity. This pain may cause considerable disruption to their normal routine, with many restricting their activities and interrupting their schooling. In the under 12s chest pain may signify organic disease but this appears to be less likely in the adolescent (Selbst 1990). Common chest pains experienced during adolescence are caused by precordial catch syndrome and hyperventilation.

Precordial catch syndrome
This is felt as 'catching' around the heart beneath the left nipple. Breathing may become shallow as the child is afraid to take a deep breath until the pain subsides. Poor posture may be a cause. The condition is not serious and disappears with time. Treatment,

especially for an anxious adolescent, includes plenty of reassurance that it is not a heart attack. Serious cardiovascular disease in this age group is an extremely rare cause of chest pain and pain would normally be felt as crushing in the centre of the chest, the pain frequently radiating down an arm.

Hyperventilation
Hyperventilation may be a cause of pain resulting from over-breathing and is often accompanied by dizziness, light-headedness and occasionally tingling in the hands and around the mouth. Again reassurance and breathing into a paper bag should control symptoms.

Resources

- Niggemann (2002) for information on functional symptoms
- Shrier et al. (2002) but, like so many guidelines, the one section that appears to be missing in this otherwise useful article is pain management

---

CHRONIC PAIN

Chronic pain in young adults does occur and can have a significant impact on their quality of life. Chronic pain will interfere with sleep, everyday activities, education and of course relationships and their wider social context.

Principles of assessment and evaluation for chronic pain

Very few tools have been designed specifically for use in older children or young adults so we do encourage you to refer to the previous chapter for a selection of tools appropriate for children and to the following chapter for tools that have been developed for use in adults. Weel et al. (2005) devised a 'pain related check-list' to measure the impact of pain in adolescents. The four main areas relate to concentration, mobility, acceptability and mood. Using the following principles should help select the most appropriate assessment tool depending on a child's condition, cognitive development, psychology, social and other factors:

- Is the pain chronic with acute flairs or just present all the time?
- Is rehabilitation the focus of the therapy?

- Will the information gathered be in the child's best interest, i.e. will enough information be obtained?
- Will too much information be gathered for the context in which it is to be used?
- Is the information specific enough for the particular child and his or her condition?

When selecting an assessment tool consider the following:

- Taking time with the child to establish a collaborative relationship
- Allowing the child to expand on formal assessment issues and to elaborate on the responses
- Actively listening to the information given
- Discussing the implication of the pain on the child's lifestyle and quality of life as far as possible

Ensure the tool will cover aspects such as pain intensity, functional capacity, mood, sleep, personality, beliefs, coping, medication and side effect monitoring and psychosocial history (Jamison 1996).

Neuropathic pain

- **Type 1 diabetes**. This is becoming more common in children. However, literature on the management of any potentially painful diabetic neuropathy in adolescents and children is sparse. See Chapter 6 for the management of this condition in adults.
- **Complex regional pain syndrome type 1**. See Chapter 4.
- **Scar pain**. The incidence of chronic scar pain is known to be surprisingly high in adults following such operations as limb amputation, thoracotomy and mastectomy (Perkins & Kehlet 2000; Macrae 2001). The incidence of scar pain in children and young adults is poorly researched. Young people are now more likely to be diagnosed with other neuropathic conditions such as complex regional pain syndrome. Previously unexplained pain in young people who have undergone surgery could be related to the development of scar pain or other surgery-related tissue damage. This may go unrecognised.

Pharmacological strategies
Minimise nociception from any underlying or ongoing injury with simple analgesia and/or opioids. Tricyclic antidepressants and anticonvulsants are the mainstay of neuropathic pain management in adults, but their relevance to children or young adults is unclear. Local anaesthetic blocks, administered by sub-cutaneous infiltration or directly to specific nerves, can produce long-lasting pain relief for some chronically painful conditions such as post-appendectomy scar pain (Rowbotham & Fields 1989; Goddard 2002). The application of a local anaesthetic patch may, in the future, prove a useful and safe strategy for pain confined to a relatively small area.

Non-pharmacological strategies
- Very careful explanation to the children and their parents is required.
- Physical therapy is vital to restore function as quickly as possible and reverse any dysfunction caused by inappropriate immobilisation that may have been occurring prior to diagnosis.
- Referral to a psychologist can be helpful to give support.
- TENS.
- Biofeedback and self-hypnosis may be helpful in particularly motivated teenagers.
- Dorsal column stimulation is sometimes offered as a last resort.

Musculoskeletal or body wall pain

Juvenile rheumatoid arthritis (JRA)
There are several different types of juvenile arthritis but juvenile rheumatoid arthritis (JRA) is the most common, affecting about 10% of children with arthritis. Systemic onset may cause inflammation of internal organs as well as pain and damage to joints. JRA can affect children at any age but is uncommon in the first 6 months of life. This condition may not immediately be diagnosed because some children may not complain of pain at first and swelling may not be immediately obvious. Limping, stiffness first thing in the morning, reluctance to use the affected limb, reduced activity and eventually fever and joint swelling are classical symptoms.

Pharmacological strategies

First-line treatment is usually an NSAID, such as ibuprofen or naproxen. As these drugs may be taken for some time additional stomach protection may be necessary. Disease-modifying antirheumatic drugs (DMARDs) are added as a second-line treatment when arthritis remains active despite NSAID therapy. DMARDs include drugs such as methotrexate and more recently 'anti-TNF agents'. Each of these medications may cause side effects that need to be monitored closely. Some of these drugs are only licensed for adults, but clinical trials are currently being conducted to test their efficacy and safety in children. In addition, new therapies are being developed all the time and will likely be available in the future. Where only a single joint is involved, a steroid may be injected before any additional medications are given. Oral steroids such as prednisalone may be used in certain situations, but only for as short a time and at the lowest dose possible. In children it is very important to avoid the long-term side effects such as weight gain, poor growth and risk of infection.

Non-pharmacological strategies

Children should be encouraged to continue attending school and participating in all the usual activities as much as possible. Adolescents especially should be encouraged to undertake social activities with their peers so they do not feel isolated and left out. A positive outlook and continued physical activity will help to prevent loss of function and increase strength and endurance. Where available a rheumatology team can assist with the complex needs of the child and family.

Fibromyalgia

Fibromyalgia causes painful muscles and fibrous tissue and is recognised as a medical condition in adults. However, juvenile fibromyalgia syndrome (JFS) appears to be very similar, with widespread persistent pain, sleep disturbance and multiple tender points. Its pathogenesis is probably related to muscle deconditioning and persistent disruption or a reduction of stage 4 sleep. There may be generalised immune activation involving several of the cytokines. The resulting prolonged inactivity from pain and fatigue may lead to further muscle deconditioning

(Buskila et al. 1993). Of children and adolescents diagnosed with chronic pain syndrome 25–40% fulfil the criteria for JFS (Schanberg et al. 1996) and the most common age for onset is between 13 and 15 years (Yunus & Masi 1985).

Pharmacological strategies
The mainstay of medication appears to be the tricyclic antidepressants. In the same way that the treatment of adult fibromyalgia using standard analgesia appears to be ineffective, so it is for children and adolescents.

Non-pharmacological strategies
Non-pharmacological strategies appear to be more effective than any of our current pharmacological therapies. They are based on education, exercise, developing proper sleeping habits, lifestyle adjustments, stress management and counselling, relaxation and cognitive-behavioural techniques. Exercise is centred on ergonomic training, postural exercise and proper body mechanics, with functional activity training to increase strength, range of motion, tolerance and pain threshold.

Resources
- Brown & Greenwood-Klein (2001) for information on juvenile fibromyalgia and the role of the occupational therapist
- Reid et al. (2005) for information on parent and child interactions and juvenile fibromyalgia and arthritis

Growing pains
Any young person complaining of pain should receive consideration and understanding. The term 'growing pains' has caused a great deal of controversy regarding the cause and definition of 'growing pain' and its prevalence (2.6–50% of children). The literature is wide-ranging – one paper suggested that some children diagnosed with depression also report 'growing pains' (McWilliams et al. 2004). Others suggest that it may be due to biomechanical foot abnormalities. The research is not clear but the message is that any child complaining of musculoskeletal pain should receive further questioning and assessment.

Visceral pain

Chest pain

Asthma, chronic bronchitis and allergic cough (especially from cigarette smoke) are typical examples of respiratory disorders sometimes responsible for chest pain. In over 45% of cases a cause for the chest pain will not be found. While children may have real pain, no medical illness is apparent. Stress is thought to be implicated in up to 75% of cases. Confident reassurance is the key and possibly a change of routine and lifestyle.

Inflammatory bowel disease

Inflammatory bowel diseases such as Crohn's disease (CD), ulcerative colitis (UC) and indeterminate colitis can be particularly distressing for adolescents. They usually have little experience of previous diseases, other than acute infections, and they will often be very reluctant to discuss their bowel function. On top of this they may well experience pain, which is a very common symptom of these conditions. Eighty eight percent of adolescents with CD and 96% of adolescents with UC will report pain as a major symptom (Kirschner 1998).

Pharmacological strategies

Drug therapy to modify the course of the disease and therefore the symptoms is currently the first-line treatment. This includes antibiotics and corticosteroids with elemental and polymeric formulas to induce and maintain remission in active CD and reverse growth failure (Kirschner 1998). Immunomodulatory agents are also used to reduce the need for steroids and hospitalisation. As with many complex disease processes, a combination therapy is recommended to control symptoms and limit drug-induced side effects. With literature on chronic and potentially painful conditions scant, attention is usually given to the management of pain in the period before drug therapy begins to reduce symptoms.

Paracetamol and opioids would appear to be the most effective treatment. Opioids may also help to reduce diarrhoea and codeine is often given for this. NSAIDs with their gastrointestinal side effects would be contraindicated, especially concurrently with steroid therapy.

Non-pharmacological strategies

The following are some of the specific complementary and alternative therapies reportedly used by adolescents with inflammatory bowel disease, as reported in a study by Day et al. (2004):

- Probiotics
- Fish oils
- Herbal remedies
- Vitamin supplements
- Homeopathy
- Relaxation
- Chiropractic
- Massage
- Aloe vera
- Evening primrose oil

How effective these particular therapies may be for this condition is still open to speculation; however, there is some evidence of an anti-inflammatory effect with fish oils (Belluzi 2002) and possibly tissue healing with glucosamine (Salvatore et al. 2000). More research needed is needed to define the exact benefits and potential side effects of complementary therapies for adolescents with inflammatory bowel disease.

Resources

- Day et al. (2004) for information on complementary and alternative medicine for inflammatory bowel disease
- Hotopf et al. (1998) for information on chronic abdominal pain
- Kirschner (1998) for information on the differences in the management of irritable bowel disease in children compared to adults
- The National Digestive Diseases Information Clearinghouse (NDDIC) is an information dissemination service of the National Institute of Diabetes and Digestive and Kidney Diseases (NIDDK). The NIDDK is part of the National Institutes of Health (NIH) in the USA: www.digestive.niddk.nih.gov/ddiseases/pubs/crohns (accessed October 2005)
- The National Association for Colitis and Crohn's Disease (NACC) is a UK organisation: www.nacc.org.uk (accessed October 2005)

Endometriosis

Although this is a disease usually associated with women over 20, it can and does begin in younger women and teenagers. It is a chronic and usually progressive disease that occurs almost exclusively in women of reproductive age. It can be extremely debilitating and to make matters worse the diagnosis is often missed, with one study alarmingly reporting up to 70% of women with endometriosis having been wrongly informed at least once that their symptoms are psychogenic in origin and 'all in their head' (Ballweg 1997). It can also impede fertility.

Endometriosis is caused by tissue normally located in the lining of the uterus as endometrium migrating to the body cavity rather than being shed with menstruation. Because this tissue is hormone-sensitive it will respond much the same as endometrium and therefore cyclically will break apart and bleed. Because this localised bleeding cannot be discharged it can cause the surrounding tissues to become inflamed, swollen and painful. The inflammation can then lead to scaring and adhesions, progressively damaging and distorting the affected organs. Symptoms include:

- Pain before and during menstruation
- Pain during or after sexual intercourse
- Infertility
- Painful urination and bowel movements during menstruation
- Diarrhoea and constipation
- Nausea
- Backache
- Ectopic pregnancy
- Abdominal bloating and cramping

Pharmacological strategies
The pharmacological management of this unpleasant condition centres on analgesia and hormonal therapy. Progestins limit the oestrogen-stimulated growth of endometrial tissues and induce atrophy. Progestin therapy has been reported to provide excellent pain relief, with uncontrolled trials indicating a pain relief rate of 90% (Luciano et al. 1988; Schlaff et al. 1990). Oral contraceptives are often prescribed to relieve dysmenorrhoea. Sometimes a weak synthetic androgen is also used for pain control. It works by shrinking implanted endometrial tissue and may have some effect on the immune system, which is also thought to be implicated in

the development of this disease. GnRH agonists are sometimes used to alter hormone balance and improve symptoms.

Analgesics centre on aspirin and other NSAIDs. Aspirin appears to be the least effective in relieving symptoms and the most likely to cause stomach upset, nausea, vomiting and ulcers (Janbu et al. 1979). Not surprisingly NSAIDs with their prostaglandin synthesis blocking properties are effective in as many as 80% of women (Milsom & Andersch 1984). Paracetamol with no significant anti-inflammatory effects is less effective (Janbu et al. 1979). Commonly used NSAIDs include naproxen, ibuprofen and mefenamic acid. Because the response to an NSAID is so individual it is often beneficial to switch to a different compound until the most effective one is found. Some patients will experience pain so severe that strong opioids may be necessary. These patients should be closely monitored and opioids should only be used in combination with other direct interventions by a specialist clinician.

Non-pharmacological strategies
Conservative surgery to remove all visible endometriosis via a laparoscope may use direct excision, diathermy or laser vaporisation. At the same time, any adhesions can be released. Unfortunately, recurrence is common. Although this would not be offered to adolescents, when symptoms are very severe the only treatment may be a total hysterectomy and bilateral oophorectomy, with the inevitable onset of menopause, a prospect that may cause a considerable degree of anxiety even in youngsters whose symptoms at present appear relatively mild.

Other popular non-pharmacological strategies include:

- Dietary changes
- Nutritional supplements such as evening primrose oil or fish oil capsules are suggested to reduce menstrual cramps with their anti-inflammatory properties
- Chinese medicine and herbal remedies
- Yoga
- Stress reduction techniques such as relaxation therapy, as prolonged stress may disrupt hormonal balance and weaken the immune function

• Gossypol derived from cottonseed has also been suggested, but safety concerns limit its investigation

Herbal products are increasingly coming under scrutiny for their safety and potential interaction with drug therapy. They should be carefully reviewed before being recommended or encouraged (Physicians' Desk Reference 1998).

Resources

See Shrier et al. (2000), Greco (2003), Laufer et al. (2003) and Holland-Hall & Brown (2004) for further information on pelvic pain and endometriosis
  The following associations have special sections for teenagers:

• The Endometriosis SHE Trust (a UK organisation): www.shetrust.org.uk (accessed October 2005)
• The Endometriosis Association (a US organisation), including the booklet *Are You a Teenager?*: www.endometriosisassn.org (accessed October 2005)

Recurrent headaches
Non-organic headaches are one of the most common somatic complaints in schoolchildren (Larsson 1991). Headache is the most extensively investigated pain complaint in non-clinical populations of children (Goodman & McGrath 1991).

Types of headache
The following are common types of headache:

• Migraine
• Episodic and chronic tension-type headaches

Migraine appears to have a strong genetic link (Goadsby 2005).

Pharmacological strategies
Paracetamol (15 mg/kg) and ibuprofen (10 mg/kg) are shown to be effective. Paracetamol was shown to be more rapid, but ibuprofen gave better overall relief (Hamalainen et al. 1997). If this fails a trial of dihydroergotamine 20–40 µg/kg is supported.

  If this fails subcutaneous sumatriptan can be as effective in children as in adults (Larsson 1995) but further study is needed. Early administration of treatment choice is advocated. Beta blockers may have some value prophylactically but more studies are needed (Hermann et al. 1995).

Non-pharmacological strategies

- Education of parents and child to encourage self management
- For migraine sufferers, learning the triggers and how to avoid these is important
- Stress management
- Cognitive-behavioural therapy
- Relaxation training
- Biofeedback
- Ensuring a good fluid intake and regular meals

Assessment for headache

There are often problems with diagnosis in children. This is based on descriptions of the headache quality and some children have difficulty providing information about several features of their headache (Wober-Bingol et al. 1995), although this should be less of a problem for older children and adolescents. Diaries are useful where children rate their pain and impairment on a scale of 0–5 or 0–10 four times daily at breakfast, lunch, in the afternoon and at bedtime, in addition to listing medication taken.

Other measures based on the diary and reported by Larsson (1999) include:

- Headache index: total weekly headache activity score based on 28 recordings per week (0–140)
- Headache-free days in a week (0–7)
- Headache frequency: number of discrete weekly headache episodes (only two per day) (0–14)
- Average headache duration: average number of recorded time points per headache episode (0–4 per day)
- Peak headache intensity: the single highest headache intensity rating per week
- Mean headache intensity: the average of all 28 headache recordings

Resources

- *Bandolier* for diagnosing migraine: www.jr2.ox.ac.uk/bandolier/booth/migraine/diagmig
- Goddard (2002) for a useful overview of the child with chronic pain
- Merlijn et al. (2003) for psychosocial factors and chronic pain

SUMMARY

As with younger children, adolescents' pain experiences have not been the focus of much study until fairly recently. What evidence there is supports the conclusion that they will often experience quite severe pain but not necessarily seek help or analgesia. Adolescents are moving through a transition period between relying on their parents and becoming responsible for their own health care and the choices they make. Although many adolescents may be influenced by the pain behaviour and management of their parents, how they develop their independence when faced with pain is not well researched. Becoming confident in their carers, being kept informed and being encouraged to make informed choices based on available evidence will help to lay the basis for improving their pain management in the future.

REFERENCES

Ballweg, M.L. (1997) Blaming the victim: the psychologizing of endometriosis. *Obstetrics and Gynaecology Clinics of North America* **24**, 441–453.

Belluzi, A. (2002) N-3 fatty acids for the treatment of inflammatory bowel diseases. *Proceedings of the Nutrition Society* **61**, 391–395.

Brown, G.T. & Greenwood-Klein, J. (2001) Juvenile fibromyalgia syndrome: the role for occupational therapists. *Australian Occupational Therapy Journal* **48** (2), 54–65.

Buskila, D., Press J., Gedalia A., Klein M., Neumann L., Boehm R. & Sukenik S. (1993) Assessment of nonarticular tenderness and prevalence of fibromyalgia in children. American Journal of Rheumatology, **20**, 368–370.

Chambers, C.T., Reid, G.J., McGrath, P.J., Finley, G.A. & Eleerton, M.L. (1997) A randomised trial of a pain education booklet; effects on parents' attitudes and postoperative pain management. Children's Health Care, **26**, 1–13.

Cohen, J.A. (2003) Treating acute posttraumatic reactions in children and adolescents. Biological Psychiatry, **53**(9), 827–833.

Colak, T., Ipek, T., Kanik, A., Ogetman, Z. & Aydin, S. (2003) Efficacy of topical nonsteroidal antiinflammatory drugs in mastalgia treatment. Journal of the American College of Surgeons, **196**(4), 525–530.

Day, A.S., Whitten, K.E. & Bohane, T.D. (2004) Use of complementary and alternative medicines by children and adolescents with inflammatory bowel disease. *Journal of Paediatrics and Child Health* **40** (12), 681–684.

Finley, G.A., McGrath, P.J., Forward, S.P., McNeill, G. & Fitzgerald, P. (1996) Parents' management of children's pain following 'minor' surgery. *Pain* **64** (1), 83–87.

Foa, E.B., Davidson, J.R.T. & Francis, A. (1999) The expert consensus vs guideline series: treatment of PTSD. *Journal of Clinical Psychiatry* **60** (Suppl 16), 12.

Franklin, G.F. & McRury, S. (2003) P434 topical aspirin for the treatment of neuropathic pain. *European Journal of Internal Medicine* **14** (Suppl 1), S154.

Gillies, M., Parry-Jones, W.L. & Smith, L.N. (1997) Postoperative pain in adolescents: a pilot study. *Journal of Clinical Nursing* **6** (1), 77–78.

Gillies, M.L., Smith, L.N. & Parry-Jones, W.L.I. (1999) Postoperative pain assessment and management in adolescents. *Pain* **79** (2), 207–216.

Goadsby, P. (2005) Headache. In: *Proceedings of 11th World Congress on Pain*, International Association for the Study of Pain, Sydney, Australia, 21–26 August.

Goddard, M. (2002) Clinical management of the child with chronic pain. *Pediatric Anesthesia* **12** (9), 839–840.

Goodman, J.E. & McGrath, P.J. (1991) The epidemiology of pain in children and adolescents: a review. *Pain* **46**, 247–264.

Hamalainen, M.L., Hoppu, K., Valkeila, E. & Santavuori, P. (1997) Ibuprofen or acetaminophen for the acute treatment of migraine in children: a double-blind, randomized, placebo-controlled, crossover study. *Neurology* **48** (1), 103–107.

Hermann, C., Kim, M. & Blanchard, E.B. (1995) Behavioural and prophylactic intervention studies of paediatric migraine: an exploratory meta-analysis. *Pain* **60**, 239–256.

Hotopf, M., Carr, S., Mayou, R., Wadsworth, M. & Wessely, S. (1998) Why do children have chronic abdominal pain, and what happens to them when they grow up? Population based cohort study. *British Medical Journal* **316** (7139), 1196–1200.

Jamison, R.N. (1996) Psychological factors in chronic pain assessment and treatment issues. *Journal of Back and Musculoskeletal Rehabilitation* **7**, 79–95.

Janbu, T., Lokken, P. & Nesheim, B.I. (1979) Effect of acetylsalicylic acid, paracetamol and placebo on pain and blood loss in dysmenorrheic women. *Acta Obstetrica et Gynecologica Scandinavica* (Suppl 87), 81–85.

Karling, M., Renstrom, M. & Ljungman, G. (2002) Acute and postoperative pain in children: a Swedish nationwide survey. *Acta Paediatrica* **91**, 660–666.

Kirschner, B.S. (1998) Differences in the management of inflammatory bowel disease in children and adolescents compared to adults. *Netherlands Journal of Medicine* **53** (6), 13–18.

Larsson, B. (1991) Somatic complaints and their relationship to depressive symptoms in Swedish adolescents. *Journal of Child Psychology and Psychiatry* **32**, 821–832.

Larsson, B. (1995) School-based treatment of recurrent headaches in adolescents. In: Wallander, J.L. & Sigel, L.J. (eds) *Behavioural Perspective on Adolescent Health*. Guildford Publications, New York.

Larsson, B. (1999) Recurrent headaches. In: McGrath, P.J. & Finley, G.A. (eds) *Chronic and Recurrent Pain in Children and Adolescents.* IASP Press, Seattle, pp. 115–140.

Laufer, M.R., Sanfilippo, J. & Rose, G. (2003) Adolescent endometriosis, diagnosis and treatment approaches. *Journal of Pediatric and Adolescent Gynecology* **16** (3), S3–S11.

Luciano, A.A., Turksoy, R.N. & Carleo, J. (1988) Evaluation of oral medrosyprogesterone acetate in the treatment of endometriosis. *Obstetrics and Gynecology* **72**, 323–327.

Macrae, W.A. (2001) Chronic pain after surgery. *British Journal of Anaesthesia* **93**, 1123–1133.

McWilliams, L., Goodwin, R.D. & Cox, B. (2004) Depression and anxiety associated with three pain conditions: results from a nationally representative sample. *Pain* **111** (1–2), 77–83.

Merlijn, V.P.B.M., Hunfeld, J.A.M., van der Wouden, J.C., Hazebroek-Kampschreur, A.A.J.M., Koes, B.W. & Passchier, J. (2003) Psychosocial factors associated with chronic pain in adolescents. *Pain* **101** (1–2), 33–43.

Milsom, I. & Andersch, B. (1984) Effect of ibuprofen, naproxen sodium and paracetamol on intrauterine pressure and menstrual pain in dysmenorrhea. *British Journal of Obstetrics and Gynaecology* **91**, 1129–1135.

Niggemann, B. (2002) Functional symptoms confused with allergic disorders in children and adolescents. *Pediatric Allergy and Immunology* **13** (5), 312–318.

Olsson, G.L. (1999) Neuropathic pain in children. In: McGrath, P.J. & Finley, G.A. (eds) *Chronic and Recurrent Pain in Children and Adolescents.* IASP Press, Seattle, pp. 75–98.

Peters, J.W.B., Bandell Hoekstra, I.E.N.G., Huijer Abu-Saad, H., Bouwmeester, J., Meursing, A.E. & Tibboel, D. (1999) Patient controlled analgesia in children and adolescents: a randomized controlled trial. *Pediatric Anesthesia* **9** (3), 235–241.

Physicians' Desk Reference (1998) *Physicians' Desk Reference (PDR) for Herbal Medicines.* Medical Economics Co., Montvale, New Jersey.

Quentin, R. & Lansac, J. (2000) Pelvic inflammatory disease: medical treatment. *European Journal of Obstetrics and Gynecology and Reproductive Biology* **92** (2), 189–192.

Reid, G.J., McGrath, P.J. & Lang, B.A. (2005) Parent–child interactions among children with juvenile fibromyalgia, arthritis, and healthy controls. *Pain* **113** (1–2), 201–210.

Robert, R., Blackeney, P.E., Villarreal, C., Rosenberg, L. & Meyer, W.J. (1999) Imipramine treatment in pediatric burn patients with symptoms of adult stress disorder. *Journal of the American Academy of Child and Adolescent Psychiatry* **38**, 873–882.

Roberts, G. (2004) A review of the efficacy and safety of opioid analgesics post-craniotomy. *Nursing in Critical Care* **9** (6), 277–282.

Romsing, J., Ostergaard, D., Drozdziewicz, D., Shultz, P. & Ravn, G. (2000) Diclofenac or acetaminophen for analgesia in paediatric tonsillectomy outpatients. *Acta Anaesthesiologica Scandinavica* **44** (3), 291–295.

Rowbotham, M.C. & Fields, H.L. (1989) Post-herpetic neuralgia: the relation of pain complaint, sensory disturbance and skin temperature. *Pain* **39**, 129–144.

Royal College of Nurses (2003) *Clinical Practice Guidelines. The Recognition and Assessment of Acute Pain in Children.* Available at www.rcn.org.uk/publications/pdf/guidelines/cpg_contents.pdf.

Salvatore, S., Heuschkel, R., Tomlin, S., et al. (2000) A pilot study of N-acetyl glucosamine, a nutritional substrate for glucosamine synthesis, in paediatric inflammatory bowel disease. *Alimentary Pharmacology and Therapeutics* **14** (12), 1567–1579.

Savedra, M., Tesler, M., Holzemer, W. & Ward, J. (1999) *Adolescent Paediatric Pain Tool (APPT) User's Manual.* College of Nursing Institute, University of California, San Francisco.

Saxe, G., Stoddard, F., Courtney, D., et al. (2001) Relationship between acute morphine and the course of PTSD in children with burns. *Journal of the American Academy of Child and Adolescent Psychiatry* **40** (8), 915–921.

Schanberg, L.E., Keefe, F.J., Lefebvre, J.C., Kredich, D.W. & Gil, K.M. (1996) Pain coping strategies in children with juvenile primary fibromyalgia syndrome: correlation with pain, physical function, and psychological distress. *Arthritis Care and Research* **9** (2), 89–96.

Schlaff, W.D., Dugoff, L., Damewood, M.D. & Rock, J.A. (1990) Megestrol acetate for treatment of endometriosis. *Obstetrics and Gynecology* **75** (4), 646–648.

Selbst, S.S. (1990) Chest pain in children. *American Family Physician* **41**, 179–186.

Shaheen, S.O., Newson, R.B., Sherriff, A., et al. (2002) Paracetamol use in pregnancy and wheezing in early childhood. *Thorax* **57**, 958–963.

Shrier, L.A., Moszczenski, S.A., Emans, S.J., Laufer, M.R. & Woods, E.R. (2002) Three years of a clinical practice guideline for uncomplicated pelvic inflammatory disease in adolescents. *Journal of Adolescent Health* **27** (1), 57–62.

Tesler, M., Savedra, M., Holzemer, W., Wilkie, D., Ward, J. & Paul, S. (1997) The word-graphic rating scale as a measure of children's and adolescents' pain intensity. *Research in Nursing and Health* **14**, 361–371.

Weel, S., Merlijn, V., Passchier, J., et al. (2005) Development and psychometric properties of a pain related problem list for adolescents (PPL). *Patient Education and Counselling* **58** (2), 209–215.

Wober-Bingol, C., Wober, C., Karwautz, A., et al. (1999) Recurrent headaches in children and adolescents. In: McGrath, P.J. & Finley, G.A. (eds) *Chronic and Recurrent Pain in Children and Adolescents.* IASP Press, Seattle, pp. 115–140.

Yang, P., Wu, M.T., Hsu, C.C. & Ker, G.-H. (2004) Evidence of early neurobiological alternations in adolescents with posttraumatic stress disorder: a functional MRI study. *Neuroscience Letters* **370** (1), 13–18.

Yunus, M.B. & Masi, A.T. (1985) Juvenile primary fibromyalgia syndrome. A clinical study of thirty-three patients and matched normal controls. *Arthritis and Rheumatism* **28** (2), 138–145.

Pain in the Middle Adult Years (18–55 Years)

6

INTRODUCTION

As we grow older all of us will have experienced the pain of a sprain, strain or maybe even a broken bone, and many of us might have had pain after surgery or labour pain giving birth. However, with increasing age we also become more vulnerable to metabolic disorders, degenerative changes and chronic illness. This chapter explores some of the commonly experienced pains of adult life.

LEARNING OBJECTIVES

❏ To describe the possible mechanisms of commonly experienced painful conditions in adults
❏ To describe psychosocial and environmental aspects of pain
❏ To outline the assessment and management of acute and chronic pain commonly experienced in adulthood
❏ To understand the importance of continuous reassessment and treatment adjustment to ensure effective pain management
❏ To describe the possible mechanisms that may increase susceptibility to the development of chronic non-malignant pain

---

Box 6.1 The prevalence of pain

Pain is very common. *Pain – There's a Lot of it About* is the title of an overview in Bandolier (1999) principally reporting on a study carried out in the Grampian region of Scotland which questioned 3,605 adults about chronic pain defined as 'pain or discomfort, that persisted continuously or intermittently for longer than three months'. Half of the respondents reported having chronic pain. This increased with age, from about one-third of those aged 25–34 to almost two-thirds in those older than 65 years. Chronic pain was associated with older age, living in rented council accommodation, being retired or being unable to work.

The above study seems to confirm earlier work suggesting that 50% of adults will experience muscle or joint pain in a year (Unruh 1996) and 80% will experience low back pain at some stage during their life (Waddell 1998).

ACUTE PAIN

Principles of assessment and evaluation for acute pain

Ideally tools should include a pain intensity score using one of the following:

- Visual analogue scale (VAS)
- Verbal rating scale
- Numerical rating scale
- Present pain intensity (PPI)

Some patients will understand and feel more comfortable with one type of rating than with another and sometimes giving patients the choice can improve pain assessment. Figure 6.1 gives an example of an acute pain assessment tool incorporated into a standard postoperative monitoring chart.

A pain assessment chart should also include an area to document the pain-relieving strategies used and analgesia given, with a column for any side effects or adverse reactions experienced to ensure these are not repeated. A body map can be a useful addition.

Present pain intensity (PPI)

This is a subscale of a far larger questionnaire – the McGill Pain Questionnaire (1975) – but has been found to be simple and easy to use for assessing the intensity of pain. It can be used as a self-report (where the patient fills it in) or it can be filled in with the health care professional. It consists of a scale of 0–5, where 0 represents 'no pain' and 5 is 'excruciating', and is classed as a 'uni-dimensional' tool as it only assesses intensity.

- 0 – No pain
- 1 – Mild
- 2 – Discomforting
- 3 – Distressing
- 4 – Horrible
- 5 – Excruciating

Like all pain assessment charts available, it will only work well when used. So often when patients are asked about their pain,

Fig. 6.1 Postoperative monitoring chart that includes pain assessment. (Reproduced with kind permission of Poole Hospital NHS Trust.)

Box 6.2 The Joint Commission on Accreditation of Healthcare Organisations (JCAHO) standards for pain and its management

- Patients have the right to recognition and control of their pain
- Thorough pain assessment of patients identified with pain
- Perform effective pain management and rehabilitation
- Educate staff, patient and family about pain
- Ongoing quality improvement of pain management

(Reproduced with permission from the Joint Commission on Accreditation of Healthcare Organisations (2000) *Joint Commission Resources Standards for Pain and its Management.* JCAHO, Oakbrook Terrace, Illinois.)

---

their report bears little or no relation to what staff have documented. Nursing assessment and documentation of pain has repeatedly been reported as inadequate. The USA has now made pain assessment mandatory if hospitals are to attain or retain accreditation. See Box 6.2 for a brief synopsis of the standards as they relate to pain management.

Surgery

The following would be common procedures undertaken on adults:

- Head and neck surgery possibly for tumour or infection
- Gynaecological surgery such as hysterectomy and caesarean section
- Upper abdominal pancreatic surgery
- Upper abdominal surgery to remove the gall bladder or undertake fundoplication for reflux (both procedures are increasingly being undertaken via a laparoscope involving short stay or day case surgery)
- Lower abdominal surgery such as hernia repair
- Bowel surgery to remove tumours, damage caused by Crohn's disease, ulcerative colitis or to repair a perforation caused by diverticulitis
- Appendicectomy
- Orthopaedic surgery to decompress nerves in carpal tunnel syndrome or repair broken bones or ligaments

Experiencing postoperative pain (short stay patients)

Case study

John has just returned to the day case unit following surgery to repair an anterior cruciate ligament. Although this can be painful, using a multimodal approach helped to ensure he was discharged that evening without significant pain or experiencing severe or unpleasant side effects.

Box 6.3 Developing chronic pain after surgery

Research suggests that chronic pain after surgery is a common and serious side effect associated with inadequately managed acute pain. Other possible contributing factors include pain preoperatively, surgical approaches that risk nerve damage, chemotherapy, radiotherapy, and psychological and depressive symptoms. Data are available for post-thoracotomy, cholecystectomy, mastectomy, hernia and amputation pain. See Bandolier (2002a).

Pharmacological strategies

Despite technological advances in anaesthesia and analgesia, reported pain levels after day surgery remain high (Coll et al. 2004). Innovative approaches are beginning to illustrate how pre-emptive and multimodal analgesia (local anaesthetic plus regular opioids with non-opioids) may reduce not only acute postoperative pain but also the incidence of chronic pain that develops in some individuals after surgery (Reuben et al. 2002; see Box 6.3).

Table 6.1 shows the outcomes of one such innovative approach designed to control surgical pain and reduce the risk of a poor long-term outcome.

Non-pharmacological strategies

Preparation for patients undergoing day case surgery may enable screening to take place to ensure greater support for those showing high levels of anxiety or fearfulness, which have been shown to correlate with increased pain and poorer outcome (Emflorgo 1999; Carr et al. 2005). Pre-assessment clinics enable staff to spend time with patients, answering questions and providing leaflets detailing what to expect following surgery for their particular condition. Information giving is a simple strategy that can routinely be incorporated into surgical care and has been shown to improve outcomes (Sjoling et al. 2003).

Resources

- Association of Anaesthetists of Great Britain and Ireland (1994)
- British Association of Day Surgery (2005)

Table 6.1 Data presented at the American Society of Regional Anaesthesia and Pain Medicine Annual Spring Meeting 2002 by Reuben et al. (2002), showing the results of pre-emptive multimodal analgesia for anterior crutiate ligament day case surgery.

Measured	Standard care (% of patients)	Multimodal care (% of patients)
Patients discharged on day of surgery	58	96
Rehab at 6 months	68	91
Knee pain at 1 year	14	4
Developed chronic pain	4	1

Experiencing postoperative pain (longer stay)

Case study

Peter, aged 52 years, was admitted to hospital to undergo an anterior resection of his colon for cancer, which went ahead without complication. Prior to surgery he was offered and accepted a thoracic epidural which not only provided analgesia during his operation but also continued into the post perative period. The epidural catheter was connected to a pump administering a solution of bupivacaine and fentanyl in 500 ml normal saline. The pump enabled experienced nursing staff to adjust the rate in order to maintain analgesia, either increasing the rate if pain was experienced or reducing the rating if pain control was good but unacceptable side effects developed. Once the epidural was discontinued on day four, Peter was able to maintain his pain control using a range of regular analgesia including non-opioids and low dose oral opioids. He was mobilising well and discharged on day five.

Pharmacological strategies

To prevent different doctors prescribing different analgesics and perhaps lower doses than required, the introduction of a preprinted 'sticky label' which can be attached to a patient's drug chart can standardise prescribing. An example of a sticky label currently used in a district general hospital for the management of all acute and trauma pain is given in Fig. 6.2. This is similar to the one devised for children, and you will see the strategy begins with paracetamol to which ibuprofen may be added if not contraindicated. It also includes both intravenous and oral morphine, which may be added if a combination of full dose, regular paracetamol and ibuprofen fail to control pain. Combining non-opioids with opioids produces a synergistic effect and has the potential to enable reduced doses of opioids to be administered, thereby reducing side effects (Kehlet & Dahl 1993). It also enables pain to be rapidly brought under control rather than risk delays, which were a common feature of previous practice.

You will notice that weak opioids, such as codeine, have been excluded. This is because evidence suggests that paracetamol and ibuprofen are both more effective than any of the weak opioids alone (Bandolier 2005). This is covered in further detail in Chapter 2. If both these analgesics have failed within a hospital setting where assessment and monitoring are conducted regularly, then it can be very useful if nurses are able to immediately titrate morphine for the rapid relief of pain. See Fig. 6.3 for an example of an algorithm to assist nursing staff in the safe and effective administration of intravenous opioids for moderate to severe pain.

Pain left inadequately controlled can and does escalate. Therefore this ability to rapidly move up the analgesic ladder can lead to a dramatic improvement in patients' experiences of pain control (Layzell 2005). It is psychologically reassuring too as staff can immediately respond to the patient's pain. See Appendix 6.1 for an example of suggested analgesia for patients in acute pain taken from an acute district hospital. The guideline is available to each ward in paper format or via the hospital's Intranet system.

When the management of acute pain is compromised because a patient has a history of substance abuse, particularly with opioids, then developing an easily accessible evidence-based

ADULTS ONLY

Signature
Date
Bleep no.   Pharmacy
V3

MORPHINE IV

IV assessed staff only
1 mg IV prn – max 10 mg
Use APS protocol for guidance
on dose and time

PARACETAMOL

Route:	Dose:	Frequency
PO/PR	1 g	QDS

IBUPROFEN

Delete if NSAID contraindicated

Route:	Dose:	Frequency
PO/SL	400 mg	TDS

ORAL MORPHINE

10 mg/5ml

Omit during epidural or PCA

Age guide:	Dose:	Frequency:
16–70 yrs	10–30 mg	3–6 hourly
>70 yrs	5–10 mg	4–6 hourly

ONDANSETRON

Route:	Dose:	Frequency:
IV/PO	4 mg	8 hourly

MAGNESIUM HYDROXIDE (Laxative)

Delete in bowel or abdominal
surgery patients

Route:	Dose:	Frequency:
PO	20–40 ml	Nocte

Fig. 6.2 Example of a sticky label printed with a range of pre-prescribed analgesia to control acute pain and medication for common potential side effects. All it needs is a doctor's signature and the date. (Reproduced with kind permission of Poole Hospital NHS Trust.)

**ALGORITHIM FOR ADMINISTRATION OF
INTRAVENOUS OPIOIDS DILUTED IN 10 ml
NORMAL SALINE**

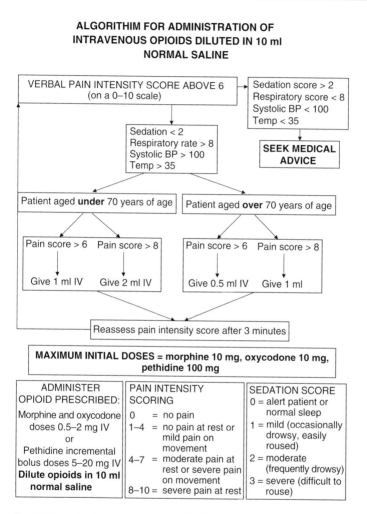

ADMINISTER OPIOID PRESCRIBED:	PAIN INTENSITY SCORING	SEDATION SCORE
Morphine and oxycodone doses 0.5–2 mg IV or Pethidine incremental bolus doses 5–20 mg IV **Dilute opioids in 10 ml normal saline**	0 = no pain 1–4 = no pain at rest or mild pain on movement 4–7 = moderate pain at rest or severe pain on movement 8–10 = severe pain at rest	0 = alert patient or normal sleep 1 = mild (occasionally drowsy, easily roused) 2 = moderate (frequently drowsy) 3 = severe (difficult to rouse)

Fig. 6.3 Example of a pain assessment tool with an algorithm that enables nurses to safely and effectively titrate intravenous opioids. (Reproduced with kind permission of Poole Hospital NHS Trust.)

guideline may help staff to manage these patients' pain more confidently and effectively. It may also help avoid some of the conflict and difficulties that can arise when managing these patients' pain, the care of whom can be complex and very challenging. Appendix 6.2 provides an example of an easy general guideline for health care professionals.

Non-pharmacological strategies

Although the evidence for some of these interventions is inconclusive (Seers & Carroll 1998) they can be helpful when used with pharmacological strategies.

- Patient information given preoperatively has been shown to be beneficial for in-patients as well as patients being discharged the same day (Sjoling et al. 2003).
- Cutaneous stimulation or transcutaneous electrical nerve stimulation (TENS) has been used effectively to reduce postoperative pain, but systematic reviews have not supported this – mainly due to poor research study design. Other interventions such as massage and touch can be helpful.
- The use of relaxation strategies and music resulted in a reduction in the perception of pain after surgery (Good et al. 2001).
- Guided imagery – talking through holiday memories of pleasant views; imagining a warm sunny day with an emphasis on the sensations of warmth, sun and the gentle sound of waves lapping on a shoreline.
- Comfort strategies such as positioning and warmth.

Nurses may not always be able to reduce the pain (if you are waiting for an anaesthetist perhaps), but by staying with the patients, understanding their pain and accepting their discomfort, a nurse can provide tremendous support at this time. Pain, anxiety and depression have also been implicated in post-operative recovery (Carr et al. 2005) and nurses need to recognise patients who are anxious or low in mood if interventions or referral are to be made.

Think about patients recovering from their surgery in a pleasant environment with a good view, television with multiple channels or the latest movies and attentive and caring staff in whom they have confidence that reports of pain will be responded to.

Now consider the person who is isolated in a side room with no visual stimulation, bored and alone and aware that if he or she is in pain and press the buzzer he/she will have a long wait before anybody responds. It is easy to see whose pain may need stronger pharmacological strategies in order to remain comfortable.

Resources

- Evidence-Based Perioperative Medicine, Geneva (2004) *The Infinite List of Systematic Reviews in Anaesthesia, Analgesia and Critical Care*: www.hcuge.ch/anesthesie/anglais/evidence/arevusyst.htm#top. Or follow the links from Bandolier's Pain site: www.jr2.ox.ac.uk/bandolier/index (accessed October 2005)
- Australian and New Zealand College of Anaesthetists and Faculty of Pain Medicine (2005)
- National Guideline Clearinghouse: *Clinical Practice Guideline for the Management of Postoperative Pain* and *Assessment and Management of Acute Pain*. Both available at www.guideline.gov (accessed October 2005)
- Sherwood et al. (2003)
- Scottish Intercollegiate Guidelines Network (2004): excellent clinical guidelines for postoperative care but sadly lacking in advice and guidelines for analgesia
- Tramer (2001a, 2001b) for controlling nausea and vomiting

Acute trauma

Injury will always result in some pain but extensive tissue damage does not necessarily result in more severe pain. Minor injuries, particularly near nerve endings, can be very painful whereas major trauma may leave patients in shock seemingly uncomplaining of the pain you would anticipate for the degree of tissue damage. Typical causes of trauma include:

- Work-related accidents
- Road traffic accidents
- Sports injuries
- Bony and soft tissue injury
- Head injury
- Spinal and neck injuries, e.g. whiplash
- Low back pain
- Burns – chemical, cold, heat
- Scalds

Experiencing acute trauma pain

Case study

Brian is a 35 year old engineer who fell from some scaffolding and has been admitted to Accident and Emergency with a compound fracture of his femur. Despite being given 10 mg of morphine IV and Entonox by the ambulance crew he is in extreme pain as he is taken into a resuscitation bay. What more could be done for him?

Pharmacological strategies

Pain exacerbates the stress response and vice versa and is aggravated by movement and transport. Keeping an injured limb immobilised will reduce initial pain. However, untreated or undertreated pain in the field can become significant pain in the Accident and Emergency department (Marcotte & Metz 2004). In this case, following pre-agreed protocols, Brian was given morphine in the ambulance for the early instigation of analgesia. In addition he was given Entonox to help control any break-through pain experienced during his journey to hospital. On arrival in the Accident and Emergency department, additional assessment of Brian's pain intensity, sedation level and respiratory rate resulted in rapid titration of further intravenous morphine to achieve optimal analgesia (Pasero 2003). Intense pain acts as an antagonist to the side effects of strong opioids such as respiratory depression and excessive sedation (McQuay 1999). Titration against side effects ensures that a therapeutic dose can be reached safely. In Brian's case he had a high tolerance to opioids, he was a large fit man who enjoyed a regular drink of alcohol and the therapeutic dose for him was closer to 25 mg of intravenous morphine before his pain was finally brought under control. A normal range of intravenous morphine for severe pain can be anywhere between 3 mg and 30 mg. He was closely monitored in the high dependency area of the Accident and Emergency department, where he remained comfortable and experienced no significant opioid side effects except a very mild feeling of sleepiness for which he was quite grateful.

As intravenous morphine can wear off within 2–6 hours, just as for children, a balanced approach should be taken; using a simple analgesic such as regular paracetamol with the addition of a regular NSAID if pain control proves problematic is a logical approach (Campbell et al. 2004). Oral opioids may still be required for breakthrough pain or on a regular basis in addition to non-opioids as part of an analgesia regime and can be given safely and effectively following simple guidelines (Gordon et al. 2004).

Each regime must be tailored to the individual's requirements as inter- and intra-individual differences in responses to both painful stimuli and analgesics are well recognised in all age groups (American Pain Society 2003). The limb must remain immobilised until permanent fixation, usually with an open reduction and fixation, can take place. In elderly patients with fractured femurs there is a move to use more local anaesthetic blocks to reduce the risks and side effects of high dose opioids. In Brian's case the higher dose of morphine brought his pain under control and postoperatively a PCA with oral non-opioids was effective.

Non-pharmacological strategies
Reassurance and calm can do much to allay fear in the initial stages of trauma. Comfort and distraction strategies will also help, as being immobilised for any length of time is unpleasant and can lead to pressure sores, osteoporosis and/or muscle atrophy as well as incredible boredom.

Resources

- *Consensus Statement of the American Society for Pain Management Nursing* and the *American Pain Society on the Use of 'As Needed' Range Orders for Opioid Analgesics in the Management of Acute Pain*. Their websites are www.aspmn.org (American Society for Pain Management Nursing) and www.ampainsoc.org (American Pain Society) (accessed October 2005)

Acute musculoskeletal or body wall pain

Experiencing acute low back pain

Case study

Jane is 42 years old and has called her General Practice surgery as she is lying in bed unable to move with severe acute low back pain following a day of gardening. She has taken a dose of 500 mg of paracetamol but is very frightened as the pain is so severe. On examination she has no 'red flags', i.e. indicators of potentially serious pathology such as progressive neurological deficit, pain at night, feeling unwell, weight loss, history of steroid use, etc. Although this has happened to her before she is too scared to move and wants to be taken to hospital.

Back pain is one of the most common reasons for seeking health care, sickness absence from work and long-term disability (incapacity benefits). Yet over 95% of back pain is not due to any serious disease and with the right treatment most patients can recover quickly (Waddell et al. 1999). Despite this fact, some individuals will go on to develop deconditioning and chronic disability in the absence of serious pathology, so early effective treatment is vital. Recommendations focus on triage to ensure that serious pathology (red flags) are not missed, with appropriate advice and confident reassurance given to the majority of patients who present with non-specific low back pain. Triage is based on the principles outlined in Box 6.4.

Pharmacological strategies
Pharmacological treatment strategies are based on the following:

- Administration of an effective analgesia sufficient to enable early mobilisation, which has taken over from the traditional and outdated advice to lie down and rest until pain subsides
- Analgesia such as regular paracetamol and/or an NSAID taken at full dose (e.g. up to 800 mg ibuprofen if necessary three times a day) and maybe an adjuvant such as a muscle relaxant

---

Box 6.4 Red flags

Diagnostic triage is the differential diagnosis between:

- Simple backache (non-specific low back pain)
- Nerve root pain
- Possible serious spinal pathology

Simple backache: specialist referral not required:

- Presentation 20–55 years
- Lumbosacral, buttocks and thighs
- 'Mechanical' pain
- Patient well

Nerve root pain: specialist referral not generally required within first 4 weeks provided resolving:

- Unilateral leg pain worse than low back pain
- Radiates to foot or toes
- Numbness and paraesthesia in same direction
- SLR (straight leg raise) reproduces leg pain
- Localised neurological signs

Red flags for possible serious spinal pathology: consider prompt referral (less than 4 weeks):

- Presentation under age 20 or onset over 55
- Non-mechanical pain
- Thoracic pain
- Past history – carcinoma, steroids, HIV
- Unwell, weight loss
- Widespread neurological symptoms or signs
- Structural deformity

Cauda equina syndrome: immediate referral:

- Sphincter disturbance
- Gait disturbance
- Saddle anaesthesia

From Clinical Standards Advisory Group (1994) and Working Backs Scotland (2005).

---

for no more than a few days if pain and muscle spasm remain severe

- Opioids are sometimes included in recommendations but the weak ones are usually just that, weak, and the stronger ones tend to induce a feeling of sedation. However, strong oral opioids such as morphine may be necessary for a day or two if non-opioid and non-pharmacological strategies are failing to provide sufficient analgesia to enable patients to get up and move.

If opioids are not matched with efforts to re-establish activity their use for simple acute back pain will remain controversial. However, in the acute stages, back pain may be very severe indeed and fail to respond to a weak opioid even in combination with non-opioids. Although there is little in the way of published research, a short course of strong opioids may restore confidence sufficiently to ensure an acute back pain sufferer starts to mobilise and participate in daily activities, possibly enabling an earlier return to work.

We have found that despite being prescribed analgesia to take regularly rather than when pain is severe, patients will often not comply with this regime advice. Consequently they do not maintain a steady state of analgesia sufficient to remain mobile. Figure 6.4 is a simple patient guideline that may help to reinforce the need for regular analgesia while pain is problematic rather than only taking it when the pain is incapacitating.

Non-pharmacological strategies
- Analgesia may be combined with other physical strategies such as heat and cool or even a massage, which may improve feelings of well-being and relaxation.
- The emphasis now needs to be on return to normal activity and work as quickly as possible, sometimes accepting that being completely 'pain free' is not yet achievable.
- Confident reassurance from all health care professionals that for the vast majority, pain such as that experienced by Jane (see case study above) is due to a minor strain and is not related to anything serious.

Well established methods of triage using a red and yellow flag system can help to reassure patients and health care professionals that serious pathology is not missed and therefore there is no need for a patient to be hospitalised. This event may in fact be counter-productive. Once in hospital patients can rapidly adopt the 'sick role', getting dressed into night clothes, having meals in bed and remaining immobile, which may contribute to delayed recovery.

INFORMATION FOR PATIENTS WITH NON-SPECIFIC LOW BACK PAIN
Advice on analgesia and treatment for mild to moderate pain

Remember to keep mobile as much as possible – activity is helpful and too much rest is not good for your condition. Ask your practice for *The Back Book*, a small booklet explaining back pain. Please follow the suggested timetable. Take the tablets regularly to prevent the pain returning

---

- Paracetamol relieves pain especially when taken **regularly**. Do not take more than 8 × 500 mg tablets in 24 hours.

- Ibuprofen relieves pain and reduces inflammation. Do not take more than 6 × 400 mg tables in 24 hours.

- The anti-inflammatory effect of ibuprofen takes a few days to develop fully.

- Take the ibuprofen tablets regularly with food. This should avoid indigestion, which is a possible side effect.

- If taking 800 mg ibuprofen try and reduce this to 400 mg after 2 days.

- Both medicines can be purchased from a pharmacy. Remember to ask for the higher strength ibuprofen 400 mg tablets initially.

- If, after taking the tablets regularly for 2 whole days the pain has not eased, then consult your doctor. After 5 days you should try to reduce the number of tablets you take, starting with the ibuprofen. You may need to obtain some 200 mg tablets and reduce the dose from 400 mg to 200 mg, three times a day.

The following table suggests timings and dosages for pain relief.

Fig. 6.4 Example of a simple patient guideline to encourage regular analgesia until musculoskeletal pain subsides. (With grateful thanks to co-contributor Pam Grant, Community Pharmacist, Poole Primary Care Trust.)

Cont'd

TIME	DAY 1	DAY 2	DAY 3	DAY 4	DAY 5
Breakfast	Paracetamol 500 mg 2 × tablets and Ibuprofen 400 mg 1 or 2 tablets	Paracetamol 500 mg 2 × tablets and Ibuprofen 400 mg 1 or 2 tablets	Paracetamol 500 mg 2 × tablets and Ibuprofen 400 mg 1 tablet	Paracetamol 500 mg 2 × tablets and Ibuprofen 400 mg 1 tablet	Paracetamol 500 mg 2 × tablets and Ibuprofen 400 mg 1 tablet
Lunch	Paracetamol 500 mg 2 x tablets and Ibuprofen 400 mg 1 or 2 tablets	Paracetamol 500 mg 2 × tablets and Ibuprofen 400 mg 1 or 2 tablets	Paracetamol 500 mg 2 × tablets and Ibuprofen 400 mg 1 tablet	Paracetamol 500 mg 2 × tablets and Ibuprofen 400 mg 1 tablet	Paracetamol 500 mg 2 × tablets and Ibuprofen 400 mg 1 tablet
Teatime	Paracetamol 500 mg 2 × tablets and Ibuprofen 400 mg 1 or 2 tablets	Paracetamol 500 mg 2 × tablets and Ibuprofen 400 mg 1 or 2 tablets	Paracetamol 500 mg 2 × tablets and Ibuprofen 400 mg 1 tablet	Paracetamol 500 mg 2 × tablets and Ibuprofen 400 mg 1 tablet	Paracetamol 500 mg 2 × tablets and Ibuprofen 400 mg 1 tablet
Bedtime	Paracetamol 500 mg 2 × tablets	Paracetamol 500 mg 2 × tablets	Paracetamol 500 mg 2 × tablets	Paracetamol 500 mg 2 × tablets	Paracetamol 500 mg 2 × tablets

Fig. 6.4 *Continued.*

The speed with which deconditioning may occur in the back is alarming and switching postural muscles on again is not always simply a matter of getting up and walking around (Young 2004).

The diagnosis and treatment of back pain has been the subject of considerable research and guideline development over the past few years, with excellent information available via the Internet. A small example of this advice is summarised in Box 6.5, listing assessments for diagnosis of acute non-specific low back pain and

---

Box 6.5 Summary of assessments for diagnosis and recommendations for treatment of acute non-specific low back pain

Assessments for diagnosis should be undertaken as follows:

- Case history should be taken and a brief examination carried out
- If history taking indicates possible serious spinal pathology or nerve root syndrome, carry out more extensive physical examination, including neurological screening when appropriate
- Undertake diagnostic triage at the first assessment as a basis for management decisions
- Be aware of psychosocial factors, and review them in detail if there is no improvement
- Diagnostic imaging tests (including X-rays, CT and MRI) are not routinely indicated for non-specific low back pain
- Reassess those patients who are not resolving within a few weeks after the first visit, or those who are following a worsening course

The following are recommendations for treatment:

- Give adequate information and reassure the patient
- Do not prescribe bed rest as a treatment
- Advise patients to stay active and continue normal daily activities, including work if possible
- Prescribe medication, if necessary, for pain relief; preferably to be taken at regular intervals; first choice paracetamol, second choice NSAIDs
- Consider (referral for) spinal manipulation for patients who are failing to return to normal activities
- Multidisciplinary treatment programmes in occupational settings may be an option for workers with subacute low back pain and on sick leave for more than 4–8 weeks

This synopsis of guidelines for the assessment and treatment of non-specific low back pain from the European Guidelines (2004) is reproduced with kind permission from the authors of the EU COST B13 programme, *European Guidelines for the Management of Acute Non-Specific Low Back Pain in Primary Care*: www.servimed.be/select/gppj/gp05210 (accessed October 2005).

---

recommendations for treatment taken from the guidelines of the European Commission Research Directorate General (2004).

Resources

- Working Backs Scotland: www.workingbacksscotland.com/index.htm (accessed October 2005)
- Faculty of Occupational Medicine: www.facoccmed.ac.uk/index.jsp (accessed October 2005)
- Arthritis and Musculoskeletal Alliance: www.arma.uk.net (accessed October 2005)
- European Commission Research Directorate General (2004)
- European Guidelines for Prevention of Low Back Pain (2004): www.back paineurope.org/web/files/wg3_guidelines.pdf#search='european%20 guidelines%20for%20prevention%20in%20low%20back%20pain' (accessed October 2005)
- Van Tulder et al. (2004): see Box 6.5 for a synopsis of assessment and treatment
- Accident Rehabilitation and Compensation Insurance Corporation of New Zealand and the National Health Committee (1997): information of risk factors for chronicity
- Abstracts of Cochrane reviews on back pain: www.cochrane.org/index0.htm (accessed October 2005)
- Van Tulder & Koes (2002)
- BMJ Clinical Evidence Series, Musculoskeletal Disorders: www.clinicalevidence.com/ceweb/conditions/msd/msd.jsp (accessed October 2005)
- Australian and New Zealand College of Anaesthetists and Faculty of Pain Medicine (2005):, Chapter 9, Specific Clinical Situations, 9.4 Acute Back Pain: www.nhmrc.gov.au/publications/_files/cp104.pdf (accessed October 2005)

Breakthrough and procedural pain

Breakthrough pain describes pain felt by patients with an underlying condition that may not be causing pain all the time, but for whom pain is a consequence of movement or an event. It may also be referred to as incident pain. Procedural pain is associated with a painful procedure such as dressing changes and is sometimes referred to as 'inflicted pain'. This is probably more accurate to describe some of the other unpleasant experiences we expose patients to, such as:

- Pain from a treatment such as venepuncture, insertion of a catheter, removal of a drain or physiotherapy
- Moving or coughing postoperatively when analgesia is suboptimal
- Constipation and defecation especially following haemorrhoids or anal surgery

- Coughing with a chest infection especially pleurisy or following trauma to the chest and ribs
- Swallowing with a sore throat
- Movement of a joint inflamed by rheumatoid arthritis
- Walking and activity bringing on ischaemic leg pain associated with intermittent claudication
- Angina pectoris as a consequence of effort, anxiety or cold

Treatment should be based on anticipating the need for pain control and ensuring patients, carers and health care staff take measures to reduce the severity of any anticipated pain by using a range of pharmacological and non-pharmacological strategies. The following are suggestions to achieve this:

- Prepare by asking patients about their previous history, for instance if they have a needle phobia or if a previous dressing change was particularly painful. For venepuncture some people may appreciate the application of a local anaesthetic cream or gel such as EMLA or Ametop gel. Alternatively some may benefit from using Entonox for short unpleasant procedures such as removal of sutures and drains.
- Warn patients in advance of physiotherapy or a dressing change and encourage them to take their regular or additional analgesia an hour or so beforehand.
- Ensure that patients postoperatively are on a regime that suits their needs and that patient controlled analgesia pumps are being used appropriately and epidural analgesia is optimised to enable patients to participate in their physiotherapy or mobilisation.
- Offer a short-acting analgesic to patients who have had haemorrhoid surgery before they go to the toilet; it might not be particularly effective but will help patients to be a little more prepared! Prevent constipation becoming an issue by encouraging patients to eat a high fibre diet, drink plenty of water and take laxatives if required.
- For patients in pain who need to cough, ensuring that adequate analgesia is established can reduce the risk of further chest complications. For example, for severe pain on coughing following fractured ribs, peripheral neural blockade may be the most helpful strategy. One block can cover the innervation of three to four ribs. Interpleural blocks can result in widespread uni-

lateral intercostal nerve block; a partial brachial plexus block and often a bilateral splanchnic nerve block are useful alternatives (Strong et al. 2002). Thoracic local anaesthetic blocks offer superior pain relief to systemic opioids alone after multiple rib fractures, thoracotomy and pancreatitis (Frenette et al. 1991).

- Reducing pain by controlling the symptoms of underlying disease, such as prescribing antibiotics to treat any infection or antispasmodics for visceral spasm, can be very helpful.
- Sucking local anaesthetic soothing lozenges or ice cubes is helpful for a sore throat.
- Applying splints, heat and cold therapy, and anti-inflammatory drugs may be helpful for inflamed joint pain. Sometimes short courses of high dose oral or intra-articular steroids are indicated for acute flares of some inflammatory conditions such as polymyalgia rheumatica (British National Formulary 2005).
- Vasodilators, beta blockers and ace inhibitors may help control the symptoms of coronary artery disease (British National Formulary 2005).
- Offering quinine to control cramp pain at night can be helpful for some patients (British National Formulary 2005).
- Lifestyle changes may also help to reduce the incidence of ischaemic and musculoskeletal pain in the long term.

Advice, reassurance, preparation and being with patients can help overcome some of the predicted pain of interventions and pain-causing pathology.

Experiencing acute breakthrough and incident pain

Case study

Polly sustained severe burns during a house fire 6 days ago. These burns have required frequent and painful redressing that initially had to be done whilst Polly was given a light general anaesthetic. Both Polly and those caring for her want to devise a plan where the dressing changes may be tolerated without a general anaesthetic, particularly as the 'nil by mouth' for several hours and then waiting for an emergency space between theatre lists is compromising her nutritional status.

Pain following severe burns is comprised of several different types: the acute pain experienced on admission, day-to-day background discomfort, pain due to surgical intervention and pain associated with dressing changes and other procedures. All need carefully planned pain relief based on regular assessment and individualised to each patient's response and tolerance.

Pharmacological strategies

The Gallagher et al. (2000) protocol describes the use of the strong intravenous opioid alfentanyl for dressing changes when pain is severe. This is a powerful opioid with a very short duration of action, which is ideal for severe procedural pain. Protocols similar to those described by Gallagher et al. using alfentanyl or offering patients conscious sedation with a combination of an anaesthetic drug such as ketamine with an anxiolytic benzodiazepine such as midazolam can provide excellent analgesia for the trauma of dressing changes (Marhofer 2001; Pees et al. 2003). However, when painful procedures are too painful for control with opioids and Entonox alone, conscious sedation is safer than a general anaesthetic (Scottish Intercollegiate Guidelines Network 2002; Department of Health 2003). Ketamine has been used for conscious sedation as it also provides pain relief and has been shown to decrease secondary hyperalgesia and increase pain thresholds better than morphine (Warncke et al. 2000). In subanaesthetic doses of up to 1 mg/kg, ketamine can also cause temporary amnesia (loss of present memory), reduce the risk of nausea and vomiting and shows no effect on respiratory depression (Schmid et al. 1999) and minimal changes in heart rate and blood pressure (White et al. 1982). The hallucinations associated with general anaesthetic doses of ketamine appear to be markedly less at these low doses and the combination of ketamine with midazolam can minimise psychotropic complications (Marhofer 2001; Pees et al. 2003).

For milder pain some patients may manage simply with an adjustment to their routine analgesia to ensure it is given prior to a dressing change and the administration of Entonox during the actual procedure. This can then be combined with non-

---

Box 6.6 Procedural pain in patients with burns

Ptacek et al. (1995), examining procedural pain in 43 patients with extensive burns, assessed pain at dressing change and found that those patients with higher pain scores reported poorer adjustment to their condition as measured by scores on the Brief Symptoms Inventory and the Sickness Impact Profile. It would seem that inadequate pain management during dressing changes affected their recovery and can have longer-term effects.

---

pharmacological strategies such as distraction, therapeutic touch, massage and music, which have been reported as beneficial (Turner 1998; Kwekkeboom 2003).

Non-pharmacological strategies
We now know that repetitive painful stimuli may lead to chronic pain syndromes (Taal & Faber 1997;Gottrup et al. 2000,) with the risk of significant psychological disturbance (Altier et al. 2002). Patients facing regular painful dressing changes are particularly vulnerable. Non-pharmacological therapies must include relevant psychological and emotional support, as patients may have to face a long recovery period, scarring and altered body image (Box 6.6). Assessment tools such as a pain diary may be helpful to chart what therapies are effective or otherwise and provide a document for others to follow that ensures strategies that are ineffective are not continually repeated.

Resources
• Allison & Porter (2004) for more information on burns pain
• Scottish Intercollegiate Guidelines Network (SIGN) (2002)

Acute visceral pain
The following is a list of common medical conditions that increase with age and are associated with acute visceral pain. Many of these conditions if left untreated will go on to become chronically painful conditions:

• Ischaemic heart disease, leading to angina pectoris, is felt as pain in the centre of the chest or radiating to the left arm and jaw, usually brought on by narrowing of the coronary arteries, aggravated by exercise, anxiety or by cold weather.

- Pancreatitis may cause severe pain associated with abscesses, cysts, calculi or tumour. Biliary tract disease and alcohol account for 80% of patients admitted to hospital with acute pancreatitis (Macpherson 1995).
- Cholecystitis is usually secondary to gall stones blocking the cystic duct and causing biliary colic as muscle fibres contract around the stone.
- Peptic ulceration of either the stomach or duodenum may cause pain particularly following the ingestion of certain substances that are known to cause irritation, such as alcohol and spicy foods.
- Crohn's disease is a chronic inflammatory disease that may occur in any part of the gut, causing acute flairs of pain. Ulcers, fistulae and granulomatous tissue can develop. The condition may be controlled with steroids, but patients will frequently experience severe pain and may ultimately require surgery. (See Chapter 5.)
- Ulcerative colitis is caused by inflammation of the first part of the large intestine, possibly resulting from an abnormal immune response to bacteria or certain foods. There is a strong familial tendency (Macpherson 1995). (See Chapter 5.)
- Tumour or a blockage in any hollow organ may lead to severe spasm pain as the organ contracts to shift the blockage or swells within the organ capsule.
- Cirrhosis of the liver results when healthy tissue is replaced by fibrous tissue similar to scarring. The liver is insensitive to pain, but swelling of the liver causes pressure on the liver capsule resulting in excruciating pain.
- Pyelonephritis describes inflammation of the kidney. It is usually caused by an infection that has spread up from the bladder or may follow a febrile disease in which bacteria leave the body via the urine. Pain is usually dull and felt as discomfort in the loins (Macpherson 1995).
- Cystitis describes inflammation of the bladder usually felt when passing urine and associated with stinging, burning and frequency. It may also be associated with a dragging ache in the lower abdomen.

Experiencing acute disease-related visceral pain

Case study

George has been admitted to the ward with acute pancreatitis. He has been given pethidine for previous bouts of pancreatitis but found that although it relieved his pain, it was effective for less than an hour. He is now rolling around the bed moaning and rates his pain as 10/10 on a numerical rating score. He is demanding increasing doses of pethidine and says it is the only drug that works.

Pharmacological strategies

The pain of pancreatitis can be very challenging to treat, especially if it has developed secondary to alcoholism. George (in the case study above) only drinks socially; however, if patients consume large quantities of alcohol or they have chronic pancreatitis treated with regular slow acting opioids, then they may be very tolerant to these drugs and require higher doses of an immediate release formulation in order to regain pain control.

There is still debate about the risk of morphine and related compounds causing both the normal and inflamed gallbladder to contract and what the relevance of this is, especially if there is any disease process involving the gall bladder or biliary tree (De Schepper et al. 2004). Morphine is still extensively used because of its longer duration of action and the fact that prescribing large doses of pethidine, which have been found to decrease gallbladder contraction (Thune et al. 1990), is problematic. Pethidine's short duration of action may lead to drug-seeking behaviour, sometimes referred to as 'pseudo addiction'. The problem is compounded by the fact that the drug can be very effective for some visceral pains. For many though it wears off far too quickly to treat anything other than transient pain. If the dose is repeated too often or a patient is given a pethidine PCA, achieving doses of 800 mg to 1 g in 24 hours is not unusual and then neurotoxicity may result (Szeto et al. 1977). In this case, giving George a morphine PCA pump may be the most effective way of ensuring he can obtain an opioid as and when required and is not undermedicated. The use of morphine is also supported by a review on the opioid analgesic effects on the sphincter of Oddi (Thompson 2001). In addition, George is given regular paracetamol for its opioid sparing and synergistic effects but will need close monitoring to ensure that morphine is not contributing to acute biliary spasm.

Unfortunately there appears to be little in the way of research into the ideal analgesia regime for painful pancreatitis, but, like any acute illness, treating the cause quickly should help to reduce pain as symptoms subside.

Non-pharmacological strategies
Giving an explanation of the reason for pain can be helpful as well as giving advice about future analgesia should the pain recur. Explaining to patients why pethidine is not used very often these days may help to reassure patients that they are getting the best available analgesia. This is especially the case if they have received this drug in the past and request it at a later date. Ongoing research may establish other opioid-related drugs as appropriate alternatives. All the previously mentioned non-pharmacological strategies can be helpful.

Resources

- National Guideline Clearinghouse (2005) has produced a guideline on the treatment of acute pancreatitis: www.guideline.gov (accessed October 2005)
- Bandolier reviews the latest evidence: www.jr2.ox.ac.uk/bandolier/index, then link to the Pain site for the section on Acute Pain (accessed October 2005)
- MedlinePlus (www.medlineplus.gov) and National Guideline Clearinghouse (www.guideline.gov) for information on ischaemic heart disease, pancreatitis, cholecystitis, peptic ulcer disease, Crohn's disease, ulcerative colitis and cystitis (accessed October 2005)
- Australian and New Zealand College of Anaesthetists and Faculty of Pain Medicine (2005): Chapter 9, Specific Clinical Situations, 9.6 Acute Medical Pain

CHRONIC PAIN

Chronic pain tends to lead to a cascade of events. Pain causes worry about damage and possible further pain, and this results in a reduction in activity levels. Reduced activity impacts on fitness, social life and the ability to earn a good living. This then has further negative consequences, with reduced fitness making

---

Box 6.7 The impact of chronic pain in the community

A postal survey conducted in Scotland found that of 4,400 patients who were randomly selected from a general practice database, 13% were moderately to severely disabled by persistent pain (Smith et al. 2001). Broad extrapolation of these figures suggests that 2–6 million people in the UK would describe themselves as having persistent, severe pain not associated with cancer.

---

it more difficult to do and enjoy activities, such as walking and gardening, that previously brought pleasure. Isolation can creep up on people as they withdraw from friends and family, and the financial consequences of being 'off sick' may start to impact on the whole family. This leads to unhelpful thoughts and beliefs such as reduced self-confidence and feelings of poor self worth. Ultimately frustration, anxiety and depression further impact on the perception of pain and the downward spiral is complete. See Box 6.7 for data suggesting that in the UK alone chronic pain and perceived disability are common in the adult population.

Helme & Gibson (2001) suggest that the principles of chronic pain management can be encapsulated in the pathophysiological basis of pain, which directs interventions toward four specific objectives:

(1) Dampen the sensitivity of nociceptors
(2) Impede the access of noxious information to the brain
(3) Alter cognitive factors underlying the perception of pain and suffering
(4) Modify behaviour, such as the overuse of medication

A further strategy, which probably needs to be included in behaviour modification programmes, is the reduction in disability and improved function. Chronic pain causes people to avoid the things they anticipate will be painful or cause further damage. Unfortunately this can lead to excessive fatigue, loss of strength, endurance and flexibility in muscles and soft tissues and ultimately further disability, social isolation, sleep difficulties and depression.

The interventions discussed above may seem straightforward but the management of chronic pain is nearly always complex, requiring strategies that can target the psychosocial consequences of unrelieved and unremitting pain as well as any pathological cause (Chapter 8 describes some of the specialist services available).

Principles of assessment and evaluation for chronic pain

Some excellent pain assessment tools have been devised specifically for chronic pain that incorporate aspects that reflect how it affects the way patients function and feel. Tools such as the short form McGill Pain Questionnaire (see Fig. 6.5) and the Brief Pain Inventory (BPI) (see Fig. 1.6) include questions to ascertain both the sensation of the pain, and how it affects function, mood and activities of daily living, and pain intensity to give an overall picture of pain. Pain diaries are also useful to capture the patients' perspective and experience of their pain. No one measure is going to be effective; rather, multiple strategies are needed including changes of diet and lifestyle as well as disease management, analgesia and adjuvant drug therapy to try to reduce the symptoms.

Assessment tools for chronic pain need to be more comprehensive than a unidimensional tool that measures just one component of the pain experience, i.e. the sensory or intensity of the pain. Unidimensional tools are appropriate for acute pain, which is treatable and usually short-lasting; they are rarely used alone for chronic pain. For chronic pain a more holistic or multidimensional assessment is required to gain a greater understanding of the nature of the pain. The McGill Pain Questionnaire is helpful as it gives a choice of words commonly used to describe pain, thus incorporating a multidimensional perspective. Patients might choose words such as 'shooting' which might suggest neuropathic pain, rather than 'throbbing' or 'aching' which could suggest an inflammatory type of pain. It is helpful for diagnostic purposes to identify the type of pain.

Brief Pain Inventory

The Brief Pain Inventory (see Fig. 1.6) is a validated and relatively quick multidimensional assessment tool that unlike the others includes a section on how pain affects daily activities. When rehabilitation is a goal, especially if pain cannot be significantly decreased, being able to improve function may ultimately improve quality of life, mood, sleep, etc. and therefore show that a therapy is beneficial even though it may not be providing an

Date: _____

Name: _____

Tick the column to indicate the level of your pain for each word, or leave blank if it does not apply to you.

	Mild	Moderate	Severe
1 Throbbing	_____	_____	_____
2 Shooting	_____	_____	_____
3 Stabbing	_____	_____	_____
4 Sharp	_____	_____	_____
5 Cramping	_____	_____	_____
6 Gnawing	_____	_____	_____
7 Hot–burning	_____	_____	_____
8 Aching	_____	_____	_____
9 Heavy	_____	_____	_____
10 Tender	_____	_____	_____
11 Splitting	_____	_____	_____
12 Tiring–Exhausting	_____	_____	_____
13 Sickening	_____	_____	_____
14 Fearful	_____	_____	_____
15 Cruel–Punishing	_____	_____	_____

Mark or comment on the above figure where you have your pain or problems.

Indicate on this line how bad your pain is — at the left end of line means no pain at all, at right end means worst pain possible.

No pain	_____	Worst possible pain

S	/33	A	/12	VAS	/10

Fig. 6.5 Short form McGill Pain Questionnaire (SF-MPQ). (Reproduced with kind permission of Prof. Ronald Melzack. Copyright R. Melzack 1975, 1984. Available at www.health-sciences.ubc.ca.whiplash.bc.pdf.mcgill1.pdf, accessed October 2005.)

improvement in perceived pain relief. Complete pain relief for a patient following a protracted period of unremitting pain may not realistically be achievable. The health care interaction should focus on gaining small reductions in pain behaviour and increases in other measurable factors such as social interaction and activity, which may be as simple as being able to hang out the washing or pick up the children again.

Neuropathic pain

Examples of neuropathic pain that becomes more common as patients begin to age are listed below:

- Trigeminal neuralgia
- Post-herpetic neuralgia
- Painful diabetic neuropathy
- Post-viral neuropathy
- Alcoholic neuropathy
- Radicular pain
- Complex regional pain syndrome
- Central pain
- Deafferentation pain
- Phantom limb pain
- Stump pain
- Pain associated with multiple sclerosis
- Pain associated with Parkinson's disease
- HIV/AIDS related pain

Most of these neuropathic pains will be dealt with in more detail in the chapter on pain in the elderly (see Chapter 7), although many of them can and do occur earlier in life. Complex regional pain syndrome has already been covered in the children's section (Chapter 4) as it is increasingly being diagnosed at an earlier age. Also on the increase appears to be neuropathic pain associated with trauma, following surgery, with the onset of diabetes, other metabolic disorders and HIV/AIDS.

The recognition of pain associated with HIV/AIDS is gaining attention. HIV/AIDS affects over 40 million people in the world and more than 49,500 in the UK (Office of National Statistics 2002). Symptoms occur as a direct and indirect consequence of the disease process and as a side effect of the antiretroviral drugs used in the treatment of the disease. Central pain and peripheral neuropathy can occur as a result of viral-mediated neurotoxicity, secondary to cellular damage (mitochondria), demyelination of nerves or low B_{12} levels. All of these have been observed in patients with HIV/AIDS. Additionally, this pain can have a substantial impact on physical performance and quality of life (Simmonds et al. 2005).

Principles of assessment and evaluation for neuropathic pain

Assessment needs to be comprehensive. Useful tools for neuropathic pain are the Brief Pain Inventory (see Fig. 1.6) and Leeds Association of Neuropathic Symptoms and Signs (LANSS) pain scale (Bennett 2001; see Appendix 6.3). Pain diaries are also helpful when no one measure is going to be effective as they enable patients and clinicians to look back on what has been used in the past and any benefit or side effects that were experienced.

Experiencing pain from diabetic neuropathy

Case study

You are working within a diabetes clinic and a patient says to you that they think they are going mad. They complain that their feet are burning up and feel unpleasantly painful. They have started to stand on the lawn at night when there is a frost on the ground as it seems to be the only thing that is giving them some relief. They cannot understand why their feet appear to look normal, although occasionally they may look a bit mottled, and why they have these very unpleasant sensations when they do not remember any injury.

Painful diabetic neuropathy is common and very unpleasant. Treatment should always be multimodal and may be particularly challenging, as analgesia alone is rarely effective. Patients will often present with co-morbidities (other ill health issues) and polypharmacy (taking more than three medications at any one time). For many years patients with this pain were particularly poorly managed, as the condition was so inadequately understood.

Neuropathic pain is felt quite differently to nociceptive pain and may actually be described more in terms of discomfort, unpleasant sensations, pins and needles, shooting pains or burning sensations. The words patients use to describe their pain are extremely important as they can indicate the type of pain they are experiencing. These unpleasant sensations may be accompanied by other problems associated with nerve damage such as loss of sensation, loss of balance, difficulty with gait and walking, maybe even foot drop as nerves become progressively more damaged and dysfunctional. Strategies to control pain need to take all these experiences into consideration as well as the effect the disease is having on the function of other organs such as the gastrointestinal tract, kidneys and heart.

Pharmacological strategies
Early intervention combined with effective treatment for the underlying disease seems to be the key. For example, improving glycaemic control in patients with diabetes may limit the development of diabetic neuropathy. Drug management for these complex pains has improved over the past 5 years. Pharmacological strategies usually start with something simple such as a trial of 1 g paracetamol taken regularly four times a day until patients reach a steady state at about 70 hours. This can then be continued if a reduction in pain is recorded over the 70 hours. If no benefit has been gained then paracetamol can be confidently discontinued as an analgesic for this condition instead of being tried again and again, often over many years. A systematic approach is essential to eliminate analgesics that are ineffective. The application of capsaicin cream derived from red-hot chilli peppers is another simple treatment, but some patients cannot tolerate the initial burning sensations associated with this cream. Tricyclic antidepressants such as amitriptyline have been used with some success for about 20 years, but side effects particularly in the elderly can severely limit their use.

In addition to the tricyclic antidepressants, gabapentin, originally developed as an antiseizure medication, is suggested, as is pregabalin. Both these drugs appear to be less toxic than the tricyclic antidepressants and trials are showing some benefit for patients with painful diabetic neuropathy (Dworkin et al. 2003). A lignocaine patch may prove a useful strategy for some patients, but usually with diabetic neuropathy the areas of pain are too large. Tramadol has a dual action on serotonin and noradrenalin reuptake (chemical messengers that form part of the pain-modulating pathway) and is also a weak opioid. Some patients may have an opioid-responsive neuropathic pain, but often the doses to treat neuropathic pain have to be higher than would normally be used, and as McQuay (1999) states this may 'raise eyebrows'! Strong long acting opioids such as slow release morphine, oxycodone controlled release or opioids such as fentanyl and buprenorphine delivered using patch technology may also find a place in treatment regimes.

Work is ongoing looking at other topical applications of certain medications such as doxepin hydrochloride (McCleane 2000), the cannabinoids (De Vry et al. 2004) and also NMDA receptor antagonists such as ketamine. NMDA receptor antagonists are sometimes used for certain types of neuropathic cancer pain, stump and phantom limb pain as well as painful diabetic neuropathy (Sang 2000; Parsons 2001; Bursztajn et al. 2004).

Non-pharmacological strategies

Non-pharmacological strategies revolve around enhancing an individual's ability to cope with pain, to increase mobility and restore function and thereby improve quality of life rather than just providing improved pain control. Many patients already employ a range of strategies that they find useful, such as cold and heat, massage, relaxation and distraction. A multimodal approach incorporating the strategies previously mentioned seems most helpful. Enhancing quality of life by patient education and confidence building are cognitive behavioural strategies that may well play a significant part (Williams et al. 1996). Restoring a good sleep pattern can be difficult if pain at night is the worst symptom, but developing a good routine may be useful. Advise patients to try to establish a regular sleep pattern – getting up at the same time every morning regardless of what time they went to bed or how badly they slept. Also advise against sleeping or catching up with a nap during the day. This may be hard at first but can re-establish a proper and lasting sleeping routine. The key message with a condition such as chronic pain, which may well be incurable, is improved self-management and self-care.

Cognitive behavioural strategies appear to have a place in the management of pain from diabetic neuropathy (Morley et al. 1999), but access to a clinical psychologist or other skilled clinician can sometimes be problematic. Electrophysical agents such as TENS may be useful for some patients, but the research is still lacking regarding this strategy. Some centres are trying spinal stimulation when all other regimes fail (Winkelmüller 1999; Nandi et al. 2004).

Resources

- National Guideline Clearinghouse of the Agency of Healthcare Research and Quality (AHRQ): www.guideline.gov (accessed October 2005)
- Bandolier: www.jr2.ox.ac.uk/bandolier/index (accessed October 2005), then link to the Pain site for information on management of specific neuropathic pains within the Chronic Non Malignant Pain section
- British Pain Society: guidelines for the use of spinal stimulation. Available at www.britishpainsociety.org (accessed October 2005)
- The Neuropathy Trust is a trust for patients, offering advice and support: www.neuropathy-trust.org (accessed October 2005)
- Finnerup et al. (2005) for an algorithm to help treat neuropathic pain

---

Chronic musculoskeletal pain

Examples of musculoskeletal pain commonly experienced in adults include:

- **Strain**: pain from a strain or sprain that fails to resolve after the normal healing time. This may be due to scarring, adhesions, as a consequence of 'wind up' or as a result of deconditioning related to psychosocial factors, some of which have been previously mentioned, such as fear avoidance and catastrophising. Typical is the development of chronic non-specific low back and neck pain. A recent article in the *New Scientist* suggested inactivity and deconditioning as possible causes of some non-specific chronic low back pain (Young 2004).
- **Joint damage**: from rheumatoid arthritis or osteoarthritis, which can cause mechanical destruction and inflammation (this is covered in more detail in Chapter 7 on the elderly).
- **Carpal tunnel syndrome**: like many chronic pain syndromes this is not fully understood but is associated with disruption within the carpal tunnel causing compression of the median nerve at the wrist (Werner & Andary 2002).
- **Fibromyalgia**: a chronic pain syndrome that predominantly afflicts women and is associated with widespread pain, tender points, insomnia and fatigue. Despite extensive research, the

etiology of fibromyalgia remains unclear although abnormal sleep patterns may be a contributing factor. There is, however, mounting evidence for central pain processing and abnormal activation of a pain-related brain region, suggesting it may be a neuropathic pain syndrome similar to complex regional pain syndrome or post herpetic neuralgia.

- **Chronic lateral epicondylalgia** (tennis elbow): describes pain usually felt on the outside (lateral) part of the elbow. Its onset is usually gradual with tenderness felt on or below the joint's bony prominence. Movements such as gripping and lifting become painful. This is thought to be caused by tiny tears in part of the tendon and muscle coverings. It may be a form of tendonitis, but if the muscles and bones are also involved, then the condition is termed epicondylitis.

- **Chronic medial epicondylalgia** (golfer's elbow): the same as tennis elbow but with the pain felt on the inside (medial) part of the elbow.

- **Bursitis** (housemaid's knee): results from inflammation of the lubricating sacs in a joint. It is not usually a chronic condition but may result from too much movement or pressure on a bursa leading to a chronic inflammation. When experienced around the wrist or ankle the condition is referred to as a ganglion.

- **Frozen shoulder**: a very painful condition of the shoulder associated with stiffness and considerable limitation of movement. It usually occurs between the ages of 50 and 70 and recovery may take many months.

- **Chronic whiplash syndrome**: may result from hyperflexion/extension injuries resulting in neck and low back pain. Like many other chronic musculoskeletal pain syndromes there is a suggestion that it may develop secondary to disuse when normal movement is restricted for a period of time.

Principles of assessment and evaluation for chronic musculoskeletal pain

Proper assessment in the early phase of the development of chronic musculoskeletal pain can improve outcome, prevent adverse effects, limit psychosocial complications and possibly reduce the risk of chronicity. The risks of developing long-term disability associated with chronic musculoskeletal pain should not be underestimated. As well as the cost in terms of personal suffering, the financial cost of chronic low back pain to the NHS and community care services alone is estimated at £1.6 billion (Maniadakis & Gray 2000) and much of this may have been avoidable if good assessment and evidence-based treatment initiatives had commenced sooner. An understanding of the impact of psychosocial factors and poor functional restoration in terms of mobility and return to work is needed by all health care professionals as well as employers.

In addition to normal pain assessment, excellent tools have been devised that help to assess a range of psychosocial variables. 'Fear avoidance' and 'catastrophising' have been found to be linked to the development of chronicity (Main & Williams 2002). These terms refer to how patients view their pain and the likelihood of these views and misconceptions adversely affecting their recovery or contributing to disability. Research has supported a multidimensional conceptualisation of pain catastrophising, comprising elements of rumination, magnification and helplessness (Sullivan et al. 2000). Knowing you have a patient at 'high risk' means you can tackle some of the negative and unhelpful thoughts and cognitions that can seriously reduce the likelihood of a successful and pain-free return to full function. As Main & Williams (2002, p. 253) state, research has shown that there are many different reasons for patients to consult their doctor with pain. They may be seeking a cure or symptomatic relief, diagnostic clarification, reassurance, 'legitimisation' of symptoms or medical certification for work absence, or to express distress, frustration or anger. Patients may also be depressed and harbour the misconception that only passive treatments will help. Unless health care professionals and employers become more aware of just how complex the development of chronic pain is they will be powerless to really help patients in a meaningful evidence-based and cost effective way.

The following is a list of some useful assessment tools and questionnaires currently available that are often incorporated into the specific management of musculoskeletal pain:

- **Questionnaires measuring disability**
  — Oswestry Disability Questionnaire (Fairbank et al. 1980)
  — Roland Questionnaire (Roland & Morris 1983)

- **Functional capacity measurement**
  - — Functional Capacity Evaluation
  - — Shuttle Walk Test
- **Beliefs**
  - — Fear Avoidance Beliefs Questionnaire (FABQ) (Waddell et al. 1993)
  - — Back Beliefs Questionnaire (BBQ) (Symonds et al. 1996)
- **Coping strategies**
  - — Coping Strategies Questionnaire (Rosenstiel & Keefe 1983)
- **Levels of distress**
  - — Distress Risk Assessment Method (Main et al. 1992; Cairns et al. 2003)
- **Measures of physical and social functioning**
  - — SF36 (Ware & Sherbourne 1992)

Chronic musculoskeletal pain is very complex as pain may be linked to a condition or trauma that has fully healed. As our understanding grows we will become more skilled in helping to predict more accurately who is most at risk of developing chronic pain. Certainly knowledge of the biopsychosocial factors associated with the development of chronic musculoskeletal pain is vital as pain following deconditioning and loss of function is difficult to reverse. As we unravel human genetics it may also become easier to predict individuals who may carry a higher inherited risk of chronicity. Early instigation of treatment in the more vulnerable may help to reduce this risk in the future.

Copers and avoiders

From good assessment it is becoming clearer that there are at least two types of chronic pain sufferer. They are listed in Box 6.8, which is taken from *The Back Book* (Roland et al. 2002), describing observations of sufferers of low back pain.

These observations could well apply to many chronic musculoskeletal pains that do not have a clear pathological basis. Strategies for treatment need to be built around a good knowledge of each individual patient. A good family GP can be vital here, though too often time to develop a relationship with and knowledge of patients and their families is in short supply.

> **Box 6.8 One who avoids activity, and one who copes**
>
> - The *avoider* gets frightened by the pain and worries about the future
> - The *avoider* is afraid that hurting always means further damage even when it doesn't
> - The *avoider* rests a lot and waits for the pain to get better
> - The *coper* knows that the pain will get better and does not fear the future
> - The *coper* carries on as normally as possible
> - The *coper* deals with the pain by being positive, staying active, or staying at work
>
> This is an extract from *The Back Book* (Roland et al. 2002) that lists observations from sufferers of low back pain. Reproduced with kind permission of the authors.

Experiencing chronic musculoskeletal pain

> **Case study**
>
> You are working in a general practice surgery in primary care and a patient presents with local pain over the lateral elbow region with spread into the forearm. The pain is intermittent, only associated with movement and is particularly aggravated by gripping objects. The pain started 16 weeks ago following a change in work activity from a clerical position to a repetitive production line job.

Pharmacological strategies

Simple analgesia such as 1 g of paracetamol four times a day is usually the first line of treatment. 'Regular' administration seems to be the key message, as often patients have tried and dismissed paracetamol in the past, but may never have reached a therapeutic steady state. If paracetamol alone fails, then if tolerated add in an NSAID or a Cox-2. Again if this fails the addition of a weak opioid is sometimes recommended, but it must be noted that weak opioids alone perform poorly and may only provide limited benefit if pain control remains inadequate on regular and full dose paracetamol and NSAID. Although it is unlikely the pain will ever be severe enough to warrant a strong opioid, in some cases a very brief trial of a low dose oral strong opioid may be sufficient to establish effective pain control and then it can be rapidly reduced or removed. The use of strong opioids for chronic non-malignant/persistent pain remains controversial and should follow evidence-based guidance. Patient and prescriber advice is available from the British Pain Society (www.britishpainsociety. org), providing a logical and rationale approach to the issue of when, where and for whom opioids may be appropriate.

Patients may benefit from a trial of additional adjuvants such as a tricyclic antidepressant if pain is beginning to impact on sleep. Depending on the diagnosis, further treatment options will vary but may include steroid injections or surgery.

Non-pharmacological strategies
Non-pharmacological strategies aim to improve strength and mobility in the arm. They initially include rest from work, heat and cold packs, exercises and maybe elastic supports or splints. Osteopathy, chiropractic or deep tissue massage may be helpful along with other physical therapies such as the Alexander technique, Pilates, Yoga or Tai Chi.

Consider the biopsychosocial impact of this pain and the influence of the workplace, particularly the impact of a repetitive, possibly boring job where employees have little control over their working day. If pain is not to return after initial treatment then working practices may have to be considered and changes negotiated with the employer similar to those suggested following the development of non-specific low back pain.

Non-pharmacological strategies for other chronic musculoskeletal pain

- Distraction, usually suggested as a strategy for acute pain, but Johnson & Petrie (1997) suggest it may also be useful for chronic low back pain and therefore possibly for other chronic musculoskeletal pain
- Hypnosis, particularly for fibromyalgia (Haanen et al. 1991) but maybe also for other chronic pain
- Exercise therapy for fibromyalgia (Richards & Scott 2002) and low back pain (Rainville et al. 2004)

- Manipulation, which has demonstrated some results in alleviating chronic low back and neck pain but is still not well established (Bronfort et al. 2004)
- Psychological treatments such as operant conditioning, classic conditioning and cognitive behavioural therapy (Roelofs et al. 2002)
- Cryotherapy with ice packs or vapocoolant spray
- Infrared therapy, typically using lamps as a heating treatment
- Laser therapy, which may selectively affect blood flow (Baxter 1994)

Resources

- Bandolier for information on management of musculoskeletal pain. Available at www.jr2.ox.ac.uk/bandolier/index, then link to the Pain site, within the Chronic Non Malignant Pain section (accessed October 2005)
- National Guideline Clearinghouse (www.guideline.gov; accessed October 2005) for guidelines on the following:
  — Carpal tunnel syndrome
  — American Academy of Orthopedic Surgeons (AAOS) clinical guideline on shoulder pain
  — Disorders of the neck and upper back
  — Disorders of the elbow
- The Cochrane Collaboration (www.cochrane.org; accessed October 2005) for helpful reviews on, for example:
  — Multidisciplinary biopsychosocial rehabilitation for neck and shoulder pain among working age adults
  — Conservative treatments for whiplash
  — Interventions for treating plantar heel pain
- National Institute of Health and Clinical Excellence (NICE) (www.nice.org.uk) or the Pain site of Bandolier (www.jr2.ox.ac.uk/bandolier/index) (both accessed October 2005) for the latest information on the appropriateness and safety of NSAIDs and Cox-2s
- MedlinePlus, a service from the US National Library of Medicine and the National Institute of Health: www.nlm.nih.gov/medlineplus/fibromyalgia (accessed October 2005)
- Fibromyalgia Association UK for information on self-help groups for fibromyalgia in the UK: www.fibromyalgia-associationuk.org (accessed October 2005)
- The National Institute of Neurological Disorders and Stroke publish some advice on the management of whiplash: www.ninds.nih.gov/index.htm (accessed October 2005)

Chronic visceral pain

Complex visceral pains are amongst some of the least well-understood chronic pain syndromes. They include:

- **Chronic pancreatitis**: presents with persistent inflammation of the pancreas that may also disrupt secretion of digestive enzymes, and the hormones insulin and glucagon. Pain can be severe, experienced in the upper abdomen, sometimes radiating to the back. It may last from hours to days, become continuous or be worsened by eating or drinking particularly alcohol. Pain management involves reducing pancreatic stimulation with a low fat diet, alleviating indigestion caused by fat, taking supplementary pancreatic enzymes, abstinence from alcohol and treating severe pain with long acting analgesia. The latter might be slow release opioids or a surgical nerve block. Surgery may be required if an obstruction is found.
- **Irritable bowel syndrome (IBS)**: may also be termed spastic colon, mucous colitis, spastic colitis, nervous stomach or irritable colon. The condition is thought to be caused by an abnormal interaction between the gut, brain and autonomic nervous system (see case study below). Symptoms can cause considerable distress and include pain, cramping, diarrhoea, bloating and constipation.
- **Interstitial cystitis**: a syndrome characterised by urinary urgency, frequency, nocturia and pain in the pelvis. It has a prevalence in the USA ranging from 10–67 per 100,000 people (Speizer et al. 1999). The symptoms of interstitial cystitis can have a profoundly disruptive effect on patients' lives and present unique challenges to physicians particularly as little appears to be known about the cause of this sometimes intense pain. Suggestions for management include treating pain aggressively (Slade et al. 1997) and yet there is little literature suggesting the ideal analgesia. Other treatment strategies suggest coating the epithelium to maintain its integrity relative to permeability with polysaccharides, which may be helpful in some patients (Parsons 1997). The impact that interstitial cystitis has on sufferers may require that in addition to effective and early pain control, appropriate referrals are made to treat depression and sexual or relationship problems. Patient edu-

cation in the absence of effective treatments strategies concerning medical, complementary/alternative and self-help strategies may well be the key to improving symptoms (Chancellor & Yoshimura 2004; Dell & Parsons 2004).

- **Endometriosis**: a condition where the cells that normally make up the lining of the uterus are found in other areas of the body. These cells are usually confined to the pelvis but can be found in the bowel or bladder, within scar tissue, within ovaries and even in the lungs. As this tissue is endometrial in origin it is under hormonal control; therefore once a month it breaks down and bleeds. Blood within the pelvis or other organs may lead to inflammation, pain and the formation of scar tissue. When occurring within an ovary it can form cysts, called 'chocolate' cysts. Self-help groups have been formed and can help patients cope with this very painful and distressing condition which also affects fertility (see also Chapter 5).

A recent publication describes pudendal neuralgia as a 'severe pain syndrome' that may complicate some painful pelvic conditions. The nerve may have become damaged or compressed by scar tissue leading to neuropathy and axonal loss, and sadly 83% of patients with this condition are misdiagnosed according to Benson & Griffis (2005). So far therapies include medical management, pudendal nerve injections, decompression surgery and neuromodulation, but more research is needed to determine the best therapy for this severe and frequently underrecognised pain syndrome.

Experiencing chronic visceral pain (IBS)

Case study

Patricia visits her general practice surgery, distressed with what she calls an acute flare of her irritable bowel syndrome, which was diagnosed when she was a teenager. She is currently experiencing significant emotional distress associated with the breakup of her marriage, the need to sell her home and the disruption caused by her two rebellious teenage daughters.

Irritable bowel syndrome (IBS) is a complex disorder of the lower intestinal tract characterised by symptoms that are often worsened by emotional stress. Although symptoms may mimic an inflammatory bowel disorder, there is an absence of any structural abnormality. The gut appears to become hypersensitive to pain, with patients experiencing altered bowel habits such as diarrhoea and/or constipation. It can occur at any age, but often begins in adolescence or early adulthood and is more common in women. Pain may be particularly felt after meals and relieved by emptying the bowel. Patients often also complain of bloating, nausea and vomiting and loss of appetite. Anticholinergic medications taken before meals, antidiarrhoea medications and quite often treatment for severe anxiety and depression including the use of low dose antidepressants tend to form the basis of symptom control.

Non-pharmacological strategies
Non-pharmacological treatment for pain is centred on relieving symptoms by changes in diet, increasing dietary fibre and possibly replacing gastrointestinal stimulants such as caffeine with herbal teas such as camomile. Other treatments aim to reduce anxiety with regular exercise and relaxation whilst improving coping strategies through increasing patients' knowledge of their condition and building self-confidence.

Resources

- National Endometriosis Society: www.endo.org.uk (accessed October 2005)
- Prodigy is a source of clinical knowledge and available evidence on common conditions and symptoms managed by primary health care professionals. Available via registration for an online password at www.prodigy.nhs.uk (accessed October 2005)
- Chronic pancreatitis: www.nlm.nih.gov/medlineplus/ency/article/000221.htm
- Interstitial cystitis: www.ic-network.com (accessed October 2005)
- MedlinePlus: www.nlm.nih.gov/medlineplus/ency/article/000246.htm (accessed October 2005)
- IBS Network, a UK self-help organisation: www.ibsnetwork.org.uk (accessed October 2005)
- International Foundation for Functional Gastrointestinal Disorders (www.iffgd.org) and Irritable Bowel Syndrome (IBS) Self Help and Support Group (www.ibsgroup.org): two USA self-help groups (both accessed October 2005)
- Main & Williams (2002): available online via the BMJ website, bmj.bmjjournals.com (accessed October 2005)

Headache and migraine

Ninety percent of all headaches are acute, resolve spontaneously and are triggered by stress or tension. Other types of headache have different triggers and are not as easily treated. Although these are included within the chronic pain section, they are usually viewed as an acute flair up of a chronic condition (see Chapter 5). The following describes the various types of headaches:

- Chronic tension headache caused by sustained tension in the muscles of the face and neck
- Migraine and cluster headaches that have a vascular origin and are characterised by intense, throbbing pain on one or both sides of the head.
- Traction headaches resulting from tension on nerves that are stretched or displaced from conditions such as squinting or brain tumours
- Inflammatory headaches caused by irritation or infection of arteries or nerves in the head, neck, ears or teeth. This pain is usually associated with an acute event such as meningitis, an inflammation of the brain's outer covering. However, headache may become persistent and chronic if associated with an arteritis (inflammation of an artery).

Principles of assessment and evaluation for headache

As patients might not actually have a headache when seeking health care, ongoing assessment may involve patients completing a pain diary to give an overview of their headache pattern. This would include keeping a record of preceding features, triggers, medication type, dose, frequency and any relief experienced in terms of complete, moderate or no relief. The following assessment tools may be useful:

- **Migraine Disability Assessment Questionnaire (MIDAS)**: to assess degree of disability experienced (Bigal et al. 2003)
- **Headache Impact Questionnaire (HIT)**: to help patients indicate the severity of their headache (Lipton 1997)
- **Headache Screening Questionnaire** (National Headache Foundation 2005)

- **Headache Needs Assessment Survey (HANA)** (Cramer et al. 2001)
- **Brief Nurse-Administered Migraine Assessment Tool** (Marcus et al. 2004)
- **Migraine Therapy Assessment Questionnaire** (Chatterton et al. 2002)

Experiencing chronic headaches

Case study

Mrs Brown aged 42 visits her GP in considerable pain as she has developed migraines and is now experiencing them regularly. This is having a negative impact on her ability to work and her enjoyment of life.

For chronic headache, assessment would need to be more comprehensive than for the occasional headache that resolves with simple analgesia and relaxation. The following would ideally be included in an initial assessment:

- Detailed history
- Functional disabilities
- Time of onset to peak (seasonal or cyclical variation)
- Frequency, duration and change
- Characteristics, e.g. pulsatile, throbbing, pressing, sharp, etc.
- Light sensitivity
- Location – unilateral, bilateral or changing
- Severity
- Precipitating or relieving features
- Pharmacological and non-pharmacological strategies tried or successful
- Aura experience (15% of migraine sufferers)
- Extracranial structures
- Neck flexion for meningeal irritation present
- Neurological examination including opthalmological examination, cranial nerve, muscle tone, sensory tone and function such as gait

For most headaches early intervention is vital before the pain can become established. Chronic headache sufferers can often predict a headache and are well placed to implement early strategies that have proved effective for them in the past. Evidence is growing that points to migraine being an inherited condition, so knowing there is a family history will also assist in diagnosis (Goadsby 2005).

Pharmacological strategies
Pharmacological strategies are based on the outcome of the assessment. For a straightforward acute headache paracetamol and/or an NSAID such as ibuprofen may be effective. For a chronic condition such as migraine, once established these analgesics may cease to be effective and the triptans may offer the best chance of pain relief (Halpern et al. 2002). Aspirin-metoclopramide is effective in the treatment of migraine with mild symptoms, parenteral metoclopramide, prochlorperazine, chlorpromazine and droperidol are effective in the treatment of acute migraine and the addition of caffeine to aspirin or paracetamol improves analgesia in acute tension-type headache (Australian and New Zealand College of Anaesthesia and Faculty of Pain Medicine 2005). Paradoxically the regular use of paracetamol and codeine has been linked to the development of chronic headaches in certain individuals (Srikiatkhachorn et al. 2000; Bahra et al. 2003).

Non-pharmacological strategies
Cognitive behavioural strategies appear to offer some benefit (Nash et al. 2004). Other strategies are not extensively studied but are said to help some migraine sufferers in the early stages before the headache becomes established. Treatment success is variable and will need to be individualised to the sufferer. The following may be useful:

- Avoid all triggers, particularly certain foods, drinks, smells, etc.
- Exercise
- Rest
- Sleep (but too much or interrupted sleep may trigger a migraine)

The following have some supporting evidence, as reviewed by Bandolier (2002b):

- Chiropractic treatment
- Feverfew
- Biofeedback
- Relaxation therapy

Resources

- Migraine Disability Assessment Questionnaire (MIDAS) website and online booklets: www.midas-migraine.net/edu/about.asp (accessed October 2005)
- Headache Impact Questionnaire (Lipton 1997)
- National Headache Foundation for educational resources available to health care professionals and patients: www.headaches.org (accessed October 2005)
- National Institute of Neurological Disorders and Stroke: www.ninds.nih.gov (accessed October 2005)
- Cochrane Collaboration for reviews of oral sumatriptan for acute migraine (www.cochrane.org/reviews/en/topics/85.html) (accessed October 2005)
- National Guideline Clearinghouse: www.guideline.gov
- Bandolier Pain site: www.jr2.ox.ac.uk/bandolier/index, under the section on Migraine
- Australian and New Zealand College of Anaesthetists and Faculty of Pain Medicine (2005). See section 9.6.5 Acute Headache.

Other common chronically painful syndromes

The following are conditions known to cause pain. Research is gradually emerging on these conditions but they remain largely poorly understood. They may well be a complex mix of psychosocial disorders, genetic disposition, impaired function and disordered perception.

- Chronic fatigue syndrome
- Somatoform disorder
- Post-traumatic stress disorders
- Anxiety disorders

SUMMARY

This chapter has explored a range of pain-eliciting diseases and events commonly associated with the middle years of life. The assessment of pain is the cornerstone of nursing care and should take place prior to the identification of suitable interventions. We encourage the selection of a range of interventions, including pharmacological and non-pharmacological approaches used in tandem to optimise the management of pain. We cannot stress enough the psychosocial impact of inadequately controlled pain during what are usually a person's most productive years.

APPENDIX 6.1
EXAMPLE OF GUIDELINES FOR PRESCRIBING ANALGESIA FOR PATIENTS IN ACUTE PAIN
(Reproduced with kind permission of Poole Hospital NHS Trust.)

Policies are available on the Intranet. The Hospital has an Acute Pain Team. There is usually a member of the team available for advice daytime Mon–Fri. Bleep XXXX or, out of hours, contact the ICU anaesthetist.

BASIC GUIDELINES
MILD/MODERATE PAIN – REGULAR Q.D.S.
PARACETAMOL and/or NSAID
MODERATE/SEVERE PAIN – as above PLUS
MORPHINE (PO, IV or PCA)

- Nurses can give IV opioids on the ward for rapid control of pain.
- Appropriate analgesia does **not** mask clinical signs or impede diagnosis. Therefore do not delay prescribing analgesia for acute pain.
- Patients on strong opioids for acute pain for more than two weeks **must** be referred to the acute pain team for assessment.
- All opioid abusers with acute pain problems should be referred to the pain team, as their management may be complex (see separate guideline on the Intranet).

Opioids: a few important points
- **First line** treatment for moderate/severe pain that has not responded to non opioid analgesia is morphine PO, IV or PCA.

- Always use Oramorph© unless the patient is nil by mouth. Analgesics by injection are **not** more effective than the appropriate titrated oral dose.
- **Avoid** IM injections.
- **All** opioids cause nausea, vomiting and constipation. Always prescribe anti-emetics and laxatives if the patient is eating.
- Reduce the dose of opioids for patients over 65 years. Morphine is cumulative in elderly patients and those with renal failure.

Oramorph© (oral morphine syrup)
- Is very effective for moderate/severe pain, particularly combined with paracetamol/NSAIDs.
- Oramorph© appears to cause fewer side effects than large doses of codeine or dihydrocodeine.
- Always prescribe **2–4 times** the effective IV morphine dose (onset usually 10–15 min).
- For persistent pain PRN opioids are often ineffective. Where pain persists, prescribe Oramorph© to be given **regularly as well as a PRN** dose and review both doses daily.
- For patients over 70 years 5–10 mg Oramorph© 6-hourly may be all that is needed, but monitor closely.
- Always prescribe a **dose range** of Oramorph© so nurses can **titrate against effect.**

Weak oral opioids
Codeine, dihydrocodeine and dextropropoxyphene are weak analgesics with many side effects. Their use (separately or in co-preparations) for initiation of analgesia for acute pain is **actively discouraged**. Use oral morphine or oxycodone for patients who need more analgesia than that provided by paracetamol ± NSAID.

Patient controlled analgesia (PCA)
Patients who are NBM and require analgesia for moderate/severe persistent pain (i.e. will need more than 2 intravenous doses) should have a PCA. Contact the Acute Pain Service **or** the on call anaesthetist **or** the Recovery Ward in theatres for advice. Please note many senior nurses in the hospital are trained to set up PCA.

Alternative opioids

- **Oxycodone** is recommended for patients who cannot tolerate morphine (i.e. morphine causes severe nausea, confusion or hallucinations). Prescribe on Acute Pain Team advice. 'Oxynorm' = short acting (4–6 hours). 'Oxycontin' = long acting (12 hours).
- **Tramadol:** as effective as paracetamol. Less sedation than morphine, but possibly more nausea/vomiting. **NOT** drug of first choice.
- **Pethidine:** Lasts 1–3 hrs at best! Toxic in large doses. Rarely used currently and is **NOT** a drug of first choice.

NSAIDs

- Very effective alone for moderate pain (especially for gynae, maxfax surgery, trauma).
- C/I in renal failure, dehydration, Hx of peptic ulcer symptoms/treatment and heart disease.
- NSAIDs reduce opioid requirement and therefore opioid side effects.
- There is little difference in efficacy or side effects of individual NSAIDs in the short term. Ibuprofen PO or S/L (melt) or diclofenac PO or PR is recommended.
- There is as yet no clear advantage for Cox-2 drugs for the short-term treatment of acute pain in healthy under 65 year olds but research and guideline development is ongoing.

For current research-based evidence on acute pain see http://www.jr2.ox.ac.uk/bandolier/booth/painpag/index.html

APPENDIX 6.2
GUIDELINES FOR MEDICAL STAFF FOR THE MANAGEMENT OF ACUTE PAIN IN OPIOID-DEPENDENT PATIENTS
(Reproduced with kind permission of Poole Hospital NHS Trust.)

Opioid-dependent patients in pain often receive inadequate opioid analgesia because of negative and judgemental staff attitudes towards these patients, unwarranted fear of overdose (underestimated opioid tolerance) and the disinhibited, aggressive or manipulative behaviour of some of these patients. These patients experience acute pain at least as much as anyone else, and there is evidence that they are actually hypersensitive to acute pain (hyperalgesia) and therefore experience MORE pain than other patients. Their pain will be easier to manage if the issue of opioid abuse is discussed openly and the planned management explained. There are two aspects of treatment.

1. Opioids for prevention of acute withdrawal
Opioid-dependent patients require **maintenance opioids** to prevent acute withdrawal syndrome, which can be dangerous in the acutely ill patient. Symptoms of withdrawal syndrome include dilated pupils, agitation, clammy skin and sweating, runny nose, nausea/vomiting, tachycardia.

2. Treatment of acute pain
Opioid-dependent patients require **larger doses** of opioids for analgesia than other patients due to pharmacodynamic tolerance and hyperalgesia.

Recommended approach
Inform the Acute Pain Service as soon as possible

- **For patients able to take ORAL drugs and who are not on a methadone programme:**
  For maintenance: Oramorph© 20–40 mg QDS
  For pain: Oramorph© 20–40 mg TWO-hourly PRN
- **For patients who are *nil by mouth*:** use a morphine PCA
  Initial loading dose (10–20 mg IV)
  Demand doses 1.5–2 mg

For patients on a methadone programme
Inform the Acute Pain Service as soon as possible

- **For patients who are able to take ORAL drugs:**
  Establish and prescribe the patient's normal daily methadone maintenance dose. This can be checked by contacting the patient's GP or pharmacist. It is usually about 30 mg/day (given in divided doses)

AND

Prescribe Oramorph© for pain: 20–40 mg PRN 2-hourly to control pain.
* **For patients who are *nil by mouth*:** use a PCA as above

Initial loading dose (10–20 mg IV) with demand doses 1.5–2 mg

Important note: for ALL patients it is impossible to accurately predict a patient's requirements. Analgesia MUST be titrated and doses reviewed regularly. Observe for symptoms of sedation, respiratory depression or withdrawal.

APPENDIX 6.3
LEEDS ASSESSMENT OF NEUROPATHIC SYMPTOMS AND SIGNS

This pain scale can help to determine whether the nerves that are carrying your pain signals are working normally or not. It is important to find this out in case different treatments are needed to control your pain.

A. Pain questionnaire
* Think about how your pain has felt over the last week
* Please say whether any of the descriptions match your pain exactly

1. Does your pain feel like strange, unpleasant sensations in your skin? Words like pricking, tingling, pins and needles might describe these sensations.
    (a) NO – My pain doesn't really feel like this   (0)
    (b) YES – I get these sensations quite a lot   (5)

2. Does your pain make the skin in the painful area look different from normal? Words like mottled or looking more red or pink might describe the appearance.
    (a) NO – My pain doesn't affect the colour of
    my skin   (0)
    (b) YES – I've noticed that the pain does make
    my skin look different from normal   (5)

3. Does your pain make the affected skin abnormally sensitive to touch? Getting unpleasant sensations when lightly stroking the skin, or getting pain when wearing tight clothes might describe the abnormal sensitivity.
   (a) NO – My pain doesn't make my skin abnormally sensitive in that area (0)
   (b) YES – My skin seems abnormally sensitive to touch in that area (3)

4. Does your pain come on suddenly and in bursts for no apparent reason when you're still? Words like electric shocks, jumping and bursting might describe these sensations.
   (a) NO – My pain doesn't really feel like this (0)
   (b) YES – I get these sensations quite a lot (2)

5. Does your pain feel as if the skin temperature in the painful area has changed abnormally? Words like hot and burning might describe these sensations.
   (a) NO – I don't really get these sensations (0)
   (b) YES – I get these sensations quite a lot (1)

B. Sensory testing

Skin sensitivity can be examined by comparing the painful area with a contralateral or adjacent non-painful area for the presence of allodynia and an altered pin-prick threshold (PPT).

1. Allodynia

Examine the response to lightly stroking cotton wool across the non-painful area and the painful area. If normal sensations are experienced in the non-painful site, but pain or unpleasant sensations (tingling, nausea) are experienced in the painful area when stroking, allodynia is present.
(a) NO – normal sensation in both areas (0)
(b) YES – allodynia in painful area only (5)

2. Altered pin-prick threshold

Determine the pin-prick threshold by comparing the response to a 23-gauge (blue) needle mounted inside a 2 ml syringe barrel placed gently on to the skin in a non-painful, and then a painful area.

If a sharp pin-prick is felt in the non-painful area, but a different sensation is experienced in the painful area e.g. none/blunt only (raised PPT) or a very painful sensation (lowered PPT), an altered PPT is present.

If a pin-prick is not felt in either area, mount the syringe onto the needle to increase the weight and repeat.

(a) NO – equal sensation in both areas (0)

(b) YES – altered PPT in painful area (3)

Scoring

Add values in parentheses for sensory description and examination findings to obtain overall score.

Total score (maximum 24):

If score <12, neuropathic mechanisms are **unlikely** to be contributing to the patient's pain

If score >12, neuropathic mechanisms are **likely** to be contributing to the patient's pain

REFERENCES

Accident Rehabilitation and Compensation Insurance Corporation of New Zealand and the National Health Committee (1997) *Guide to Assessing Psychological Yellow Flags in Acute Low Back Pain: Risk Factors for Long-term Disability and Work Loss.* Available at www.acc.co.nz/acc-publications/pdfs/ip/psychosocial-guide.pdf, accessed October 2005.

Allison, K. & Porter, K. (2004) Consensus of the pre hospital approach to burn patient management. *Accident and Emergency Nursing* **12** (1), 53–57.

Altier, N., Malenfant, A., Forget, R. & Choinière, M. (2002) Long-term adjustment in burn victims: a matched control study. *Psychological Medicine* **32** (4), 677–685.

American Pain Society (APS) (2003) *Principles of Analgesic Use in the Treatment of Acute Pain and Cancer Pain.* APS, Glenview, Illinois.

Association of Anaesthetists of Great Britain and Ireland (1994) *Day Case Surgery, The Anaesthetist's Role in Promoting High Quality Care.* Available at www.aagbi.org/pdf/daycase9.pdf, accessed October 2005.

Australian and New Zealand College of Anaesthesia and Faculty of Pain Medicine (2005) *Acute Pain Management: Scientific Evidence,* 2nd edn. Available at www.nhmrc.gov.au/publications/_files/cp104.pdf, accessed October 2005.

Bahra, A., Walsh, M., Menon, S. & Goadsby, P.J. (2003) Does chronic daily headache arise de novo in association with regular use of analgesics? *Headache* **43** (3), 179–190.

Bandolier (1999) *Pain – There's a Lot of it About.* Available at www.jr2.ox.ac.uk/bandolier/band70/b70-3, accessed October 2005.

Bandolier (2002a) *Chronic Pain After Surgery.* Available at www.jr2.ox.ac.uk/bandolier/band103/b103-4, accessed October 2005.

Bandolier (2002b) Migraine Special Issue. Available at www.jr2.ox.ac.uk/bandolier/extraforbando/migspec.pdf.

Bandolier (2005) *Analgesic League Tables.* www.jr2.ox.ac.uk/bandolier/booth/painpag/acutrev/analgesics/leagtab, accessed October 2005.

Baxter, D.G. (1994) *Therapeutic Lasers: Theory and Practice.* Churchill Livingstone, Edinburgh.

Bennett, M. (2001) The LANSS Pain Scale: the Leeds assessment of neuropathic symptoms and signs. *Pain* **92** (1–2), 147–157.

Benson, J.T. & Griffis, K. (2005) Pudendal neuralgia, a severe pain syndrome. *American Journal of Obstetrics and Gynecology* **192**, 1663–1668.

Bigal, M.E., Rapoport, A.M., Lipton, R.B., Tepper, S.J. & Sheftell, F.D. (2003) Assessment of migraine disability using the Migraine Disability Assessment (MIDAS) Questionnaire: a comparison of chronic migraine with episodic migraine. *Headache: the Journal of Head and Face Pain* **43** (4), 336–342.

British Association of Day Surgery (2004) *The Discharge Process and the Assessment of Fitness for Discharge* and *Integrated Care Pathways for Day Surgery Patients.* Available at www.bads.co.uk, accessed October 2005.

British National Formulary (2005) *British National Formulary 2005.* Available at www.bnf.org/bnf/noframes, accessed October 2005.

Bronfort, G., Mitchell Haas, D.C., Roni, M.A., Evans, L. & Bouter, L.M. (2004) Efficacy of spinal manipulation and mobilization for low back pain and neck pain: a systematic review and best evidence synthesis. *The Spine Journal* **4** (3), 335–356.

Bursztajn, S., Rutkowski, M.D. & Deleo, J.A. (2004) The role of the N-methyl-D-aspartate receptor NR1 subunit in peripheral nerve injury-induced mechanical allodynia, glial activation and chemokine expression in the mouse. *Neuroscience* **125** (1), 269–275.

Cairns, M.C., Foster, N.E., Wright, C.C. & Pennington, D. (2003) Level of distress in recurrent low back pain population referred for physical therapy. *Spine* **28** (9), 953–959.

Campbell, P., Dennie, M., Dougherty, K., Iwaskiw, O. & Rollo, K. (2004) Implementation of an ED protocol for pain management in triage at a busy level 1 trauma centre. *Journal of Emergency Nursing* **30** (5), 431–438.

Carr, E.C.J., Thomas, V.J. & Wilson Barnett, J. (2005) Patient experiences of anxiety depression and acute pain after surgery: a longitudinal perspective. *International Journal of Nursing Studies* **42** (5), 521–530.

Chancellor, M.B. & Yoshimura, N. (2004) Treatment of interstitial cystitis. *Urology* **63** (3, Suppl 1), 85–92.

Chatterton, M.L., Lofland, J.H., Shechter, A., et al. (2002) Reliability and validity of the migraine therapy assessment questionnaire. *Headache: The Journal of Head and Face Pain* **42** (10), 1006–1015.

Clinical Standards Advisory Group (1994) *Back Pain.* Department of Health, London.

Coll, A.M., Ameen, J.R.M. & Mosely, L.G. (2004) Reported pain after day surgery: a critical literature review. Integrative literature reviews and meta-analysis. *Journal of Advanced Nursing* **46** (1), 53–65.

Cramer, J.A., Silberstein, S.D. & Winner, P. (2001) Development and validation of the Headache Needs Assessment (HANA) survey. *Headache: The Journal of Head and Face Pain* **41** (4), 402–409.

Dell, J.R. & Parsons, C.L. (2004) Multimodal therapy for interstitial cystitis. *Journal of Reproductive Medicine* **49** (3), 243–252.

Department of Health (2003) *Guidelines for Conscious Sedation in the Provision of Dental Care.* Available at www.dh.gov.uk/consultations/closedconsultations/closedconsultationsarticle/fs/en?content_id=4016907&chk=gqursa, accessed October 2005.

De Schepper, H.U., Cremonini, F., Park, M.I. & Camilleri, M. (2004) Opioids and the gut: pharmacology and current clinical experience. *Neurogastroenterology and Motility* **16**, 383–394.

De Vry, J., Kuhl, E., Franken-Kunkel, P. & Eckel, G. (2004) Pharmacological characterization of the chronic constriction injury model of neuropathic pain. *European Journal of Pharmacology* **491** (2–3), 137–148.

Dworkin, R.H., Backonja, M., Rowbotham, M.C., et al. (2003) Advances in neuropathic pain: diagnosis, mechanisms, and treatment recommendations. *Archives of Neurology* **60** (11), 1524–1534.

European Commission Research Directorate General (2004) *Low Back Pain: Guidelines for its Management.* Available at www.backpaineurope.org, accessed October 2005.

Fairbank, J.C.T., Mbaot, J.C., Davies, J.B. & O'Brien, J.P. (1980) The Oswestry low back pain disability questionnaire. *Physiotherapy* **66**, 271–273.

Finnerup, N.B., Otto, M., McQuay, H.J., Jensen, T.S. & Sinrup, S.H. (2005) Algorithm for neuropathic pain treatment: an evidence based proposal. *Pain* **118** (3), 289–305.

Frenette, L., Boudreault, D. & Guay, J. (1991) Interpleural analgesia improves pulmonary function after cholesystectomy. *Canadian Journal of Anaesthesia* **38** (1), 71–74.

Gallagher, G., Rae, C.P., Kenny, G.N.C. & Kinsella, J. (2000) The use of a target-controlled infusion of alfentanil to provide analgesia for burn dressing changes. A dose finding study. *Anaesthesia* **55** (12), 1159–1163.

Goadsby, P. (2005) Headache. In: *Proceedings of 11th World Congress on Pain*, 21–26 August, IASP, Sydney, Australia.

Good, M., Stanton-Hicks, M., Grass, J.A., et al. (2001) Relaxation and music to reduce postsurgical pain. *Journal of Advanced Nursing* **33** (2), 208–215.

Gordon, D.B., Dahl, J., Phillips, P., et al. (2004) The use of 'as needed' range orders for opioid analgesics in the management of acute pain: a consensus statement of the American Society for Pain Management Nursing. *Pain Management Nursing* **5**, 53–58; also available in *Acute Pain Service Bulletin* **14** (4).

Gottrup, H., Andersen, J., Arendt-Nielsen, L. & Jensen, T.S. (2000) Psychophysical examination in patients with post-mastectomy pain. *Pain* **87** (3), 275–284.

Haanen, H., Hoendredos, H., van Romunde, L., et al. (1991) Controlled trial of hypnotherapy in the treatment of refractory fibromyalgia. *Journal of Rheumatology* **18**, 72–75.

Halpern, M.T., Lipton, R.B., Cady, R.K., Kwong, W.J., Marlo, K.O. & Batenhorst, A.S. (2002) Costs and outcomes of early versus delayed migraine treatment with sumatriptan. *Headache* **42** (10), 984–990.

Helme, R.D. & Gibson, S.J. (2001) The epidemiology of pain in elderly people. *Clinics in Geriatric Medicine* **17** (3), 417–431.

Johnson, M.H. & Petrie, S.M. (1997) The effects of distraction on exercise and cold pressor tolerance for chronic low back pain sufferers. *Pain* **69** (1–2), 43–48.

Joint Commission on Accreditation of Healthcare Organisations (2000) *Joint Commission Resources Standards for Pain and its Management*. JCAHO, Oakbrook Terrace, Illinois.

Kehlet, H. & Dahl, J.B. (1993) The value of 'multimodal' or 'balanced analgesia' in postoperative pain treatment. *Anaesthesia and Analgesia* **77**, 1048–1056.

Kwekkeboom, K.L. (2003) Music versus distraction for procedural pain and anxiety in patients with cancer. *Oncology Nursing Forum* **30** (3), 433–440.

Layzell, M. (2005) Improving the management of postoperative pain. *Nursing Times* **101** (26, 28), 34–36.

Lipton, R.B. (1997) Headache Impact Questionnaire. *Headache, the Newsletter of ACHE* **8** (3). Available at www.achenet.org/articles/54.php, accessed October 2005.

Macpherson, G. (ed.) (1995) *Black's Medical Dictionary*, 38th edn. A & C Black, London.

Main, C.J. & Williams, A. (2002) Clinical review. ABC of psychological medicine. Musculoskeletal pain. *British Medical Journal* **7** (325), 534–537.

Main, C.J., Wood, P.L., Hollis, S., Spanswick, C.C. & Waddell, G. (1992) The distress and risk assessment method. A simple patient classification to identify distress and evaluate the risk of poor outcome. *Spine* **17** (1), 42–52.

Maniadakis, A. & Gray, A. (2000) The economic burden of back pain in the UK. *Pain* **84**, 95–103.

Marcotte, A. & Metz, M. (2004) Pain management in the prehospital setting. *Journal of Emergency Nursing* **30** (5), 403.

Marcus, D.A., Kapelewski, C., Jacob, R.G., Rudy, T.E. & Furman, J.M. (2004) Validation of a brief nurse-administered migraine assessment tool. *Headache: The Journal of Head and Face Pain* **44** (4), 328–332.

Marhofer, P. (2001) Ketamine for rectal premedication in children. *Anaesthesia and Analgesia* **92**, 62–65.

McCleane, G. (2000) Topical application of doxepin hydrochloride, capsaicin and a combination of both produces analgesia in chronic human neuropathic pain: a randomized, double-blind, placebo-controlled study. *British Journal of Clinical Pharmacology* **49** (6), 574–579.

McQuay, H. (1999) Opioids in pain management. *The Lancet* **353**, 2229–2232.

Morley, S., Eccleston, C. & Williams, A. (1999) Systematic review and meta-analysis of randomized controlled trials of cognitive behaviour therapy and behaviour therapy for chronic pain in adults, excluding headache. *Pain* **80** (1–2), 1–13.

Nagi, H. (2004) Acute pain services in the United Kingdom. *Acute Pain* **5** (3–4), 89–107.

Nandi, D., Yianni, J., Humphreys, J., et al. (2004) Phantom limb pain relieved with different modalities of central nervous system stimulation: a clinical and functional imaging case report of two patients. *Neuromodulation* **7** (3), 176–183.

Nash, J.M., Park, E.R., Walker, B.B., Gordon, N. & Nicholson, R.A. (2004) Cognitive-behavioral group treatment for disabling headache. *Pain Medicine* **5** (2), 178–186.

National Headache Foundation (2005) *Headache Screening Questionnaire*. Available at www.headaches.org.

Office of National Statistics (2002) HIV Infections: By Year of Diagnosis and Route of Transmission. Available at www.statistics.gov.uk/cci/nugget.asp?id=654, accessed October 2005.

Parsons, C.G. (2001) NMDA receptors as targets for drug action in neuropathic pain. *European Journal of Pharmacology* **429** (1), 71–78.

Parsons, C.L. (1997) Epithelial coating techniques in the treatment of interstitial cystitis. *Urology* **49** (5), 100–104.

Pasero, C. (2003) Pain in the emergency department. Withholding pain medication is not justified. *American Journal of Nursing* **103**, 73–74.

Pees, C., Haas, N.A., Ewert, P., Berger, F. & Lange, P.E. (2003) Comparison of analgesic/sedative effect of racemic ketamine and S(=)-ketamine during cardiac catheterization in newborns and children. *Pediatric Cardiology* **24** (5), 424–429.

Ptacek, J.T., Patterson, D., Montgomery, B. & Heimbach, D. (1995) Pain, coping, and adjustment in patients with burns: preliminary findings from a prospective study. *Journal of Pain and Symptom Management* **10** (6), 446–455.

Rainville, J., Hartigan, C., Martinez, E., Limke, J., Jouve, C. & Finno, M. (2004) Exercise as a treatment for chronic low back pain. *The Spine Journal* **4** (1), 106–115.

Reuben, S.S., Gutta, S.B., Tarasenko, V., Steinberg, R.B. & Sklar, J. (2002) Preemptive multimodal analgesia for ACL surgery. In: *Proceedings of 27th Annual Spring Meeting and Workshops*, 25–28 April, American Society of Regional Anaesthesia and Pain Medicine, Chicago.

Richards, S.C.M. & Scott, D.L. (2002) Prescribed exercise in people with fibromyalgia: parallel group randomised controlled trial. *British Medical Journal* **325** (7357), 185–187.

Roelofs, J., Boissevain, M.D., Peters, M.L., de Jong, J.R. & Vlaeyen, J.W.S. (2002) Psychological treatments for chronic low back pain: past, present and beyond. *Pain Reviews* **9** (1), 29–40.

Roland, M. & Morris, R. (1983) A study of the natural history of back pain. Part 1: development of a reliable and sensitive measure of disability in low back pain. *Spine* **8**, 141–144.

Roland, M., Waddell, G., Klaber Moffett, J., Burton, K. & Main, C. (2002) *The Back Book*, 2nd edn. The Stationery Office, London.

Rosenstiel, A.K. & Keefe, F.J. (1983) The use of coping strategies in chronic low back pain patients: relationship to patient characteristics and current adjustment. *Pain* **17** (1), 33–44.

Sang, C.N. (2000) NMDA-receptor antagonists in neuropathic pain. *Journal of Pain and Symptom Management* **19** (1), 21–25.

Schmid, R.L., Sandler, A.N. & Katz, J. (1999) Use and efficacy of low-dose ketamine in the management of acute postoperative pain: a review of current techniques and outcomes. *Pain* **82** (2), 111–125.

Scottish Intercollegiate Guidelines Network (2002) *Safe Sedation of Children Undergoing Diagnostic and Therapeutic Procedures. A National Clinical Guideline. Scotland*. Available at www.sign.ac.uk/guidelines/fulltext/58/index, accessed September 2005.

Scottish Intercollegiate Guidelines Network (2004) *Post Operative Management in Adults. A Practical to Postoperative Care for Clinical Staff*. Available at www.sign.ac.uk/pdf/sign77.pdf, accessed October 2005.

Seers, K. & Carroll, D. (1998) Relaxation techniques for acute pain management: a systematic review. *Journal of Advanced Nursing* **27** (3), 466–475.

Sherwood, G.D., McNeill, J.A., Starck, P.L. & Disnard, G. (2003) Changing acute pain management outcomes in surgical patients – research. Available at www.findarticles.com/p/articles/mi_m0fsl/is_2_77/ai_98134862, accessed October 2005.

Simmonds, M.J., Novy, D. & Sandoval, R. (2005) The differential influence of pain and fatigue on physical performance and health status in ambulatory patients with human immunodeficiency virus. *Clinical Journal of Pain* **21** (3), 200–206.

Sjoling, M., Nordahl, G., Olofsson, N. & Asplund, K. (2003) The impact of preoperative information on state anxiety, postoperative pain and satisfaction with pain management. *Patient Education and Counselling* **51** (2), 169–176.

Slade, D., Ratner, V. & Chalker, R. (1997) A collaborative approach to managing interstitial cystitis. *Urology* **49** (5), 10–13.

Smith, B.H., Bourne, D.M., Squair, J., Philips, P.O. & Chambers, W.A. (2001) The impact of chronic pain in the community. *Family Practice* **18**, 292–299.

Speizer, E., Hunter, D.G., Curhan, S.G. & Stampfer, M.J. (1999) Epidemiology of interstitial cystitis: a population based study. *Journal of Urology* **161**, 549–553.

Srikiatkhachorn, A., Tarasub, N. & Govitrapong, P. (2000) Effect of chronic analgesic exposure on the central serotonin system: a possible mechanism of analgesic abuse headache. *Headache* **40** (5), 343–350.

Strong, J., Unruh, A.M., Wright, A. & Baxter, G.D. (2002) *Pain: Textbook for Therapists*. Churchill Livingstone, Edinburgh.

Sullivan, M.J.L., Sullivan, D., Tripp, W., Rodgers, W. & Stanish, W. (2000) Catastrophizing and pain perception in sports participants. *Journal of Applied Sport Psychology* **12**, 151–167.

Symonds, T.L., Burton, A.K., Tillotson, K.M. & Main, C.J. (1996) Do attitudes and beliefs influence work loss due to low back trouble? *Occupational Medicine (Oxford)* **46** (1), 25–32.

Szeto, H.H., Inturrisi, C.E., Houde, R., Saal, S., Cheigh, J. & Reidenberg, M.M. (1977) Accumulation of norperidine, an active metabolite of meperidine, in patients with renal failure or cancer. *Annals of Internal Medicine* **86**, 738–741.

Taal, L.A. & Faber, A.W. (1997) Burns injuries, pain and distress: exploring the role of stress symptomatology. *Burns* **23** (4), 288–290.

Thompson, D.R. (2001) Narcotic analgesic effects on the sphincter of Oddi: a review of the data and therapeutic implications in treating pancreatitis. *American Journal of Gastroenterology* **96** (4), 1266–1272.

Thune, A., Baker, R.A., Saccone, G.T., Own, H. & Toouli, J. (1990) Differing effects of pethidine and morphine on human sphincter of Oddi motility. *British Journal of Surgery* **77**, 992–995.

Tramer, M.R. (2001a) A rational approach to the control of postoperative nausea and vomiting: evidence from systematic reviews. Part

1. Efficacy and harm of anti-emetic interventions and methodological issues. *Acta Anaesthesiologica Scandinavica* **45**, 4–13.

Tramer, M.R. (2001b) A rational approach to the control of postoperative nausea and vomiting: evidence from systematic reviews. Part II. Recommendations for prevention and treatment, and research agenda. *Acta Anaesthesiologica Scandinavica* **45**, 14–19.

Turner, J. (1998) The effect of therapeutic touch on pain and anxiety in burn patients. *Journal of Advanced Nursing* **28** (1), 10–20.

Unruh, A.M. (1996) Gender variations in clinical pain experience. *Pain* **65**, 123–167.

Unruh, A.M., Ritchie, J.A. & Merskey, H. (1999) Does gender affect appraisal of pain and pain coping strategies? *Clinical Journal of Pain* **15**, 31–40.

Van Tulder, M.W. & Koes, B.W. (2002) Low back pain and sciatica: chronic. *Clinical Evidence* **8**, 1171–1187. Available at www.clinicalevidence.com, accessed October 2005.

Van Tulder, M., Becker, A., Bekkering, T., et al. (2004) *European Guidelines for the Management of Acute Nonspecific Low Back Pain in Primary Care*. EU Cost B13 Programme. Available at www.servimed.be/select/gppj/gp05210.htm, accessed October 2005.

Waddell, G. (1998) *The Back Pain Revolution*. Churchill Livingstone, Edinburgh.

Waddell, G., Newton, M., Henderson, I., Somerville, D. & Main, C.J. (1993) A Fear Avoidance Beliefs Questionnaire (FABQ) and the role of fear-avoidance beliefs in chronic low back pain and disability. *Pain* **52**, 157–168.

Waddell, G., McIntosh, G., Hutchinson, A., Feder, G. & Lewis, M. (1999) *Low Back Pain Evidence Review*. Royal College of General Practitioners, London.

Ware, J.J. & Sherbourne, C.D. (1992) The MOS 36-item short-form health survey (SF-36). I. Conceptual framework and item selection. *Medical Care* **30**, 473–483.

Warncke, T., Stubhaug, A. & Jorum, E. (2000) Preinjury treatment with morphine or ketamine inhibits the development of experimentally induced secondary hyperalgesia in man. *Pain* **86** (3), 293–303.

Werner, R.A. & Andary, M. (2002) Carpal tunnel syndrome: pathophysiology and clinical neurophysiology. *Clinical Neurophysiology* **113** (9), 1373–1381.

White, P.F., Way, W.L. & Trevor, A.J. (1982) Ketamine: its pharmacology and therapeutic uses. *Anaesthesiology* **56**, 119.

Williams, A.C. de C., Pither, C.E., Richardson, P.H., et al. (1996) The effects of cognitive-behavioural therapy in chronic pain. *Pain* **65** (2), 282–283.

Winkelmüller, W. (1999) Neuromodulation techniques in the treatment of chronic painful diseases. *Pain Reviews* **6** (3), 23, 203–209.

Young, E. (2004) TV is a switch-off for back muscles. *New Scientist* **2462** (August), 10.

Pain in Older Adults   7

INTRODUCTION

Ageing does not necessarily lead to chronic pain, but it is estimated that between 33% and 50% of people over 65 years do experience chronic pain (Harstall 2003) and within nursing home residents it can be anywhere between 37 and 80% (Ferrell et al. 1995; Allcock et al. 2002). A large population survey in the UK revealed that whilst increasing age in the elderly is not associated with overall change in the prevalence of pain, the pattern of pain prevalence in different body regions does change (Thomas et al. 2004). Although older people expect to get pain, in reality far less actually do (Helme et al. 1992). The prevalence of some types of pains such as headache, migraine, abdominal and back pain may actually decrease in these later years (Strong et al. 2002). However, cancer is far more prevalent in the elderly and this is nearly always associated with pain that is inadequately controlled (Foley 1994). Cleeland et al. (1994) found that sufferers of metastatic cancer who were aged over 70 years of age were the least likely to receive adequate analgesia for their pain. Knowledge about older people and their experience of pain is important as demographic patterns reveal a large and increasing ageing population (see Box 7.1). The aim of this chapter is to understand the unique needs of older people experiencing pain and the principles of effective pain management.

Box 7.1 Changing demographics

There were 19.8 million people aged 50 and over in the UK in 2002. This represents a 24% increase over four decades, from 16.0 million in 1961. The number is projected to increase by a further 37% by 2031, when there will be close to 27 million people aged 50 and over. (From Office for National Statistics 2002.)

LEARNING OBJECTIVES

❏ To understand the physiological and psychosocial changes that impact on the perception of pain in the older person

❏ To identify factors that might influence an accurate pain assessment in the older person

❏ To be able to select a minimum of three interventions to manage pain in the older person with acute or chronic pain.

ACUTE PAIN

Laboratory studies seem to suggest that pain perception in older people decreases with age, but once pain is felt, older people report the same severity and quality as younger people (Helme & Gibson 2001). Changes might be accounted for through alteration in nociception as well as an increase in stoicism (Gibson & Helme 2001). It is worth noting that many research studies exclude people older than 75 and thus we have little data available to help us see the pattern of pain in the older adult (Jakobsson & Hallberg 2002). A small study reviewing hospital admissions for 129 patients in their 90s revealed that gastrointestinal conditions were the most common reason (40%) for admission, with abdominal pain which settled occurring in 23 patients (16%) (Burns-Cox et al. 1997).

Principles of assessment and evaluation for acute pain

The principles of pain assessment are similar to those outlined in previous chapters, but there are special considerations for older people. As stated earlier, impaired hearing or vision as well as cognitive changes can make assessment more challenging. There is considerable evidence that pain in the older person is poorly assessed and managed (Closs 1994) and requires special strategies for accurate assessment and appropriate management (Acute Pain Management Guidelines Panel 1992). Older people may have additional co-morbidity, e.g. angina, respiratory disease or dementia. These factors may present barriers to assessment and are given special consideration at the end of the chapter. Undertaking accurate pain assessment to identify the possible cause of the pain remains essential, especially identifying the words chosen by patients to describe their pain (see Box 7.2).

Box 7.2 Older people's pain, staff perceptions and pain management

A study in Sweden interviewed 52 nursing auxiliaries, registered nurses, physiotherapists and occupational therapists in order to explore their perceptions of older people in persistent pain and the day-to-day management of their pain. Staff perceived older people as a diverse group – some complained and some did not. This would affect the interventions they offered. The authors suggest that reflective discussion on feelings related to these differing experiences of pain should be offered. (See Blomqvist 2003.)

Box 7.3 A comparison of five pain assessment scales

Five different pain assessment scales were randomly presented to older people with different levels of cognitive impairment who resided in nursing homes ($n = 113$). These included the verbal rating scale, horizontal numerical rating scale, faces pictorial scale, color analogue scale and mechanical visual analogue scale. Using the verbal rating scale was the most successful with this group, completed by 80.5% overall and 36% of those with severe cognitive impairment. (See Closs et al. 2004.)

Use an assessment tool that is easy to complete, timely and demonstrates validity and reliability. There have been several studies evaluating the use of pain assessment tools in older people (see Box 7.3). The following text gives examples of a couple of scales that might be helpful for the assessment of acute pain as well as some tools developed for assessment of acute pain in the cognitively impaired.

Present pain intensity (PPI)

A good choice of pain assessment tool is the numerical verbal descriptor, consisting of a scale of 0–5, where 0 represents 'no pain' and 5 is 'excruciating' (or it can be 0–10). There is some evidence that the elderly may find a verbal descriptor scale easiest to use (Herr & Mobily 1993). Others suggest the numerical rating scale is best (Kassalainen & Crook 2004).

There are several advantages for older people using this type of scale:

- They usually find them easy to understand.
- Some people prefer to use words rather than numbers for pain.
- Teaching patients to use them is relatively quick and easy.

- Scores are simple and easy to document.
- The tool can be read out by the nurse or carer, thus overcoming difficulties due to visual impairment.

Visual analogue scale (VAS)

Research contains conflicting advice regarding this tool for the elderly, with some studies suggesting that the VAS (see Fig. 1.3) is considered a reliable, sensitive and valid method of assessing the intensity of acute pain (Dalton & McNaull 1998), while others suggest that older people might have difficulty understanding and completing the scale (Gagliese & Melzack 1997; Gagliese & Katz 2003). Increasing age has been associated with a higher frequency of incorrect responses to the VAS (Jensen et al. 1986). A study by Herr & Mobily (1993) suggested that the elderly may find a vertical rather than a horizontal line to be more appropriate.

It is essential to understand that the word used to describe pain by one person may not have the same meaning to another and each person's report of his or her pain is individual, for example, hurt, discomfort or aching. Other tools such as 'the faces' have been criticised as being demeaning for older people. Where possible, use one of the above tools unless there is a degree of cognitive impairment.

Pain scales when cognitive impairment is an issue

The Abbey pain scale (see Fig. 7.1)

This scale was developed in order to provide an easy-to-use tool for use in residential care homes for patients suffering from acute, acute on chronic or chronic pain (Abbey et al. 2004). It was developed with residents suffering dementia who were unable to articulate their needs.

Pain Assessment Tool in Confused Older Adults (PATCOA)

PATCOA was devised in order to assess acute pain in confused older adults by observing the display of non-verbal pain cues and the level of acute confusion.

How to use scale: While observing the resident, score questions 1 to 6.
Name of resident:...
Name and designation of person completing the scale:...................
Date:.................................... **Time:**..
Latest pain relief given was... **at** .... **hrs.**

Q1. Vocalisation
 e.g. whimpering, groaning, crying   Q1 ☐
 Absent 0   Mild 1   Moderate 2   Severe 3

Q2. Facial expression
 e.g. looking tense, frowning, grimacing, looking
 frightened   Q2 ☐
 Absent 0   Mild 1   Moderate 2   Severe 3

Q3. Change in body language
 e.g. fidgeting, rocking, guarding part of body,
 withdrawn   Q3 ☐
 Absent 0   Mild 1   Moderate 2   Severe 3

Q4. Behavioural change
 e.g. increased confusion, refusing to eat, alteration
 in usual patterns   Q4 ☐
 Absent 0   Mild 1   Moderate 2   Severe 3

Q5. Physiological change
 e.g. temperature, pulse or blood pressure outside
 normal limits, perspiring, flushing or pallor   Q5 ☐
 Absent 0   Mild 1   Moderate 2   Severe 3

Q6. Physical changes
 e.g. skin tears, pressure areas, arthritis, contractures,   Q6 ☐
 previous injuries
 Absent 0   Mild 1   Moderate 2   Severe 3

Add scores for 1 – 6 and record here ▭⇒ Total pain score ☐

Now tick the box that matches the
total pain score ⇒

0 – 2	3 – 7	8 – 13	14 +
No pain	**Mild**	**Moderate**	**Severe**

Finally, tick the box which matches
the type of pain ⇒

Chronic	Acute	Acute on chronic

Fig. 7.1 The Abbey pain scale. (Reproduced with kind permission of Dr. J. Abbey, Department of Nursing, Queensland, Australia, j.abbey@qut.edu.au.)

Box 7.4 Pain assessment in patients with severe dementia

Using interviews with patients who could not report pain this study (Manfredi et al. 2003) evaluated nine patients with senile dementia and leg ulcers, using video tapes to assess the reliability and validity of facial expressions as pain indicators. Patients were videoed before and after dressing changes and this footage was shown to nurses and doctors to elicit their views on the presence or absence of pain based on their observations of facial expression and vocalisations. The study concluded that clinical observations of facial expression and vocalisation were accurate indicators for assessing the presence of pain but not intensity in patients unable to communicate because of advanced dementia.

Observable pain behaviours are an important supplement to pain assessment (see Box 7.4). We will explore these in more detail later in the section on chronic pain, reviewing additional assessment tools that consider facial expression, body language and physiological changes in more depth. These become important when cognitive impairment may limit the utility of a unidimensional verbal or visual analogue scale (Simons & Maiabar 1995; Manfredi et al. 2003).

Resources

- City of Hope Pain/Palliative Care Resource Centre: www.cityofhope.org/prc/elderly.asp (accessed October 2005)
- World Health Organization (2004): excellent 'questions and answers' about pain management
- Herr (2002) and Bird (2005) for further articles on assessing pain in older people

---

Surgery

The following would be common procedures undertaken on elderly patients:

- The surgical removal of tumours or palliative surgery
- Joint replacements such as the knee or hip
- Minor surgeries for inguinal hernia repair or tooth extraction

Experiencing postoperative pain (short stay patients)

Case study

Martin is in his late 60s, lives alone but is generally active and in good health. He was admitted to the Day Case Unit for surgery to repair an inguinal hernia. He is very independent and was keen to get home the same day. His surgery was uncomplicated but pain following his hernia repair was moderate to severe for several days. Despite advice he was reluctant to take analgesia as recommended in case he masked any 'damage' from doing too much.

Pharmacological strategies

As for all short stay patients, careful assessment immediately after surgery is vital to ensure that pain control is effective and any side effects are minimised or treated. The elderly are especially vulnerable to the side effects of analgesia; therefore certain considerations are needed. In some cases analgesia doses may have to be reduced and even halved if close observation is suggesting sedation is becoming problematic.

Provided they have normal liver function, 1 g of paracetamol is usually safe in the elderly. NSAIDs have to be given with caution, but if there are no contraindications then ibuprofen or diclofenac should be safe if taken for a short period of time, with advice given on potential side effects such as abdominal pain. Recent concerns regarding NSAIDs and the elderly and additional data on paracetamol are covered in more detail in the next section.

Although the data available suggest good efficacy of full dose codeine with paracetamol, in our experience the elderly will still experience central side effects sometimes greater than those experienced with a low dose of a strong opioid. Oxycodone appears to be a more gentle opioid in the elderly. It is available as a longer acting byphasic preparation (with immediate release and slow release properties combined). When carefully titrated to pain, it does not appear to contribute significantly to sedation, nausea and hallucinations quite like morphine does (Reuben et al. 2002).

Many elderly patients are still prescribed weak opioids such as codeine and dihydrocodeine as take-home medication following day surgery. The elderly have often taken these drugs in the past and if they have experienced poor pain control with them, then it is unlikely they will obtain significant benefit following surgery. They also run the risk that large and ineffective doses of weak opioids may lead to severe constipation, which is particularly problematic. A low dose of oral morphine (10 mg) with paracetamol may be more effective than a large dose of codeine with paracetamol but data are currently lacking. Oral morphine syrup is available in 10 mg plastic vials, which may reduce risk of accidental overdose, and as a take-home medication it is not a controlled drug and may only need to be issued to cover the first 24 hours. Alternatively longer acting oxycodone 5–10 mg b.i.d. may be useful and better tolerated. It is effective with an NNT (numbers needed to treat) of 2.2 for 5 mg immediate release oxycodone with 500 mg paracetamol. Its main drawback for day case surgery is that oxycodone is a controlled drug. Further studies are needed to see whether a one-off dose of extended release oxycodone given once prior to discharge with non-opioid analgesia on a regular basis for a few days would provide sufficient analgesia without the need to take home further strong opioids.

Patients undergoing inguinal hernia repair are often given an ilio-inguinal block, which can be very effective. However, the block will usually wear off rapidly once patients are home and then pain can be severe and take them by surprise. Patients must be warned about this and given advice about when to take medication. Older patients may present several barriers that might prevent them taking regular analgesics and nurses need to be aware of these, as follows:

- Stoicism
- Reluctance to take analgesia, fearing the drugs will do them harm, unaware of the potential long-term damage of under-treated pain (e.g. inducing chronic pain)
- Under-reporting of pain because it is what they expect to experience
- They may have had previous experiences of poor pain management and feel that there is nothing that can be done (Ferrell 1996)
- Altered hearing, speech or cognition can impede communication

They will need careful cognitive assessment to ensure they can fully understand and remember advice given especially regarding the detrimental effects of pain.

Older people ideally need to have a good support network at home to enable early discharge – someone available to collect them from hospital, stay with them for a few days and ensure that all their needs are catered for until they are able to resume their independence. It is a good idea to ensure this other person is also given advice on medication for pain control supported by a take-home information leaflet. With an ageing population good support mechanisms at home may become harder to maintain so elderly day case patients who are alert, pain free and self-caring will become a greater priority. Future analgesia development may need to concentrate on slow release compounds or longer lasting local analgesics to ensure that adequate pain relief with minimal side effects can be achieved. Currently work is being undertaken on analgesia regimens including drugs such as gabapentin prior to surgery to enhance pain control and reduce opioid requirement, which may make pain control safer for the elderly in the future (Dierking et al. 2004)

Experiencing postoperative pain (longer stay patients)

Case study

Mary is 82 years old and has developed a bowel obstruction secondary to a slow growing inoperable tumour in her abdomen. Although prior to becoming ill she was alert and leading a reasonably active and independent life within a sheltered accommodation complex, she suffers from moderate heart disease and also has mild dementia. Following major surgery her pain has appeared to be well managed with a thoracic epidural. However, assessment has been problematic as the physiological stress of surgery has caused Mary to become more confused than usual. Although her behaviour, especially when being moved, indicates that her pain control may be less than optimal, when asked by staff if she is in pain, she forgets to mention it was severe on movement and whilst lying still she just smiles and says she is fine.

Potential effects of unrelieved postoperative pain after surgery from which the elderly are particularly vulnerable include the following:

- Respiratory dysfunction (limited ability to take deep regular intakes of breath)
- Renal dysfunction
- Infection
- Delirium and confusion
- Functional impairment and impaired ambulation
- Deconditioning
- Gait disturbances
- Falls
- Slow rehabilitation
- Chronic post-surgical pain
- Depression

Pharmacological strategies

Any pain-relieving strategies may be complicated by the challenges of effective assessment in the cognitively impaired elderly patient and the fact that heart disease and other co-morbidities may be present. Caution has to be taken with patients dependent on a wide range of medications, as some of these may interact with analgesia. The mainstay of multimodal analgesia, paracetamol, plus or minus an NSAID or Cox-2, plus or minus an opioid may have to be revised. Recent evidence has indicated that NSAIDs and Cox-2 are contraindicated for patients with heart disease and opioids may only be tolerated in very low doses in the elderly. The elderly are particularly sensitive to some opioid metabolites, especially the metabolites of morphine, codeine and diamorphine when renal function is poor. These patients may benefit from an opioid with a less active metabolite such as oxycodone or methadone, which can be difficult to titrate, or fentanyl, which does not appear to produce active metabolites (Dean 2004).

Based on advice from the American Medical Association (2005), caution with any drugs in the elderly should be taken due to:

- Decreased renal function
- Decreased volume of distribution because of decreased lean body weight
- Decreased liver mass and hepatic blood flow

- Decreased activity of some drug-metabolising enzymes
- Decreased serum protein concentrations
- Decreased pulmonary function

Paracetamol

This has been assessed in the elderly and tests showed no statistical difference in the incidence of gastrointestinal adverse events between paracetamol and placebo (Langman et al. 1994; Fries & Bruce 2003). A study by Bannwarth et al. (2001) looked at multiple dosing of paracetamol in a very elderly sample of patients (84–95 year olds) taking multiple medications and found no significant drug accumulation, suggesting that paracetamol remains safe even in the very elderly. Declining organ function increased the risk of potential adverse drug effects.

Additional factors that need particular consideration in the elderly are as follows:

- Beware of exceeding maximum doses inadvertently as combination analgesic preparations and 'co drugs' already contain paracetamol.
- Paracetamol has a ceiling beyond which higher doses just risk toxicity.
- Take care when administering paracetamol to patients taking warfarin as over-anticoagulation has been reported (Hylek et al. 1998).
- Chronic or excessive use of paracetamol may impair renal function and cause hepatoxicity.
- Use cautiously in patients with alcoholism and liver disease.

NSAIDs

Serious gastrointestinal (GI) toxicity from NSAID use can occur without warning and is estimated to have led to 100,000 hospitalisations and 16,000 deaths annually in the USA and around 2,500–3,000 deaths in the UK (Blower et al. 1997; Moore & Phillips 1999; Bandolier 2005), mostly in the elderly population. Henry et al. (1993), Langman et al. (1994) and Kennedy & Small (1997) all demonstrated the risk of gastropathy increasing linearly with age, especially in the over 60s suffering with concomitant disease states and taking multiple drug therapy. Consequently elderly patients who take NSAIDs are five times more likely to die from a GI bleed as those who do not (Griffin et al. 1988). Piroxicam was associated with high risk and ibruprofen and diclofenac with lower risk (Henry et al. 1993; Langman et al. 1994; Hernandez-Diaz & Rodriguez 2000).

Renal complications may also be significant in this age group especially when good hydration is compromised. Renal excretion declines with age leading to the half-life of NSAIDs becoming longer. NSAIDs can also contribute to renal impairment by lowering the glomerular filtration rate through its antiprostaglandin effect; therefore doses should be based on the extent of hepatic or renal impairment.

Cox-2 inhibitors

These were introduced on the premise that they have comparable efficacy and anti-inflammatory properties but produced significantly less GI ulcers (Emery et al. 1999; Silverstein et al. 2000; Goldstein et al. 2003; Leese et al. 2003). NICE (2004) guidelines state that a Cox-2 inhibitor should be carefully considered in elderly patients (65 years and over) receiving NSAIDs for chronic conditions such as osteoarthritis and rheumatoid arthritis.

Recent studies have also demonstrated that there may be an increased risk of cardiovascular (CV) events in patients treated with Cox-2 inhibitors (Hippisley Cox & Coupland 2005). The VIGOR (Vioxx Gastrointestinal Outcomes Research) study established a statistically significant increased risk of cardiovascular events in the rofecoxib (now withdrawn from use) group compared to naproxin (Bombardier et al. 2000). Naproxin has been demonstrated to have a significant antiplatelet effect comparable to that of aspirin (FDA Advisory Committee 2001); therefore it is not currently clear whether the adverse results for rofecoxib were due to a signficant antithrombic effect of naproxin. This is confounded by the problem that many study participants are excluded from clinical trials because they have multiple co-morbidities and severe disease – the very category into which many elderly patients fall – so studies do not necessary reflect the realities of clinical practice.

It is probably unlikely that the adverse effects in the elderly in terms of gastrointestinal or cardiac related events are significant when NSAIDs or Cox-2s are only given for a couple of days, at a reduced dose postoperatively, in carefully selected well hydrated patients as part of a regime of multimodal therapy. However, given the research that is being undertaken and the potential risks involved, any recommendations will need to be reviewed on a regular basis. Of course some patients may wish to continue taking NSAIDs, even when they know the risks, in order to reduce their pain.

Current contraindications for NSAIDs in over 65 year old patients include a previous clinical history of gastrodudodenal ulcer, gastrointestinal bleeding or perforation, deranged renal function, clotting abnormalities, aspirin-sensitive asthmatics, low blood pressure or low urine output (less than 0.5 ml/kg per hour). NSAIDs may interact with other drugs that are highly bound to plasma proteins resulting in a potentiation of the effect of both drugs.

Opioids

Morphine appears to remain currently the drug of choice for the elderly. It has a high lipid solubility and therefore a large volume of distribution, resulting in an increased half-life. It is important to start with a low dose and titrate upwards slowly, being aware of the differing opioid requirements in the elderly (Aubrun et al. 2002). The elderly may also experience a greater analgesic effect than younger patients due to the increased sensitivity of the brain to some opioids. Extreme caution is required when opioids are administered to the elderly who may be dehydrated or hypovolaemic.

When pain is expected to continue for some time after surgery, or indeed is associated with surgery that was only palliative, long-term opioids may be required once non-parenteral pain control has been effectively established. Excessive doses or the premature use of a long-acting opioid in the opioid-naive older patient can cause over-sedation, confusion or delirium. Short-acting immediate release morphine or the slightly longer acting extended release oxycodone with an immediate release preparation for breakthrough pain can be used to titrate to an effective dose with the least side effects. Good quality data on the use of low dose opioids such as oral morphine or oxycodone have been lacking, but clinical experience confirms the value of these preparations in the elderly over weak opioids such as codeine.

It is likely that the future will emphasise the use of regional anaesthesia and combinations of a low dose strong opioid with paracetamol and possibly the inclusion of other adjuvant drugs at low doses for their opioid sparing effects.

The following is some general information on other commonly used opioids for postoperative pain.

- **Fentanyl.** This short-acting opioid is frequently used to provide perioperative analgesia as well as in continuous epidurals and as an alternative to morphine in PCAs, especially when renal function is compromised. It is also available in a patch for chronic pain management[1].
- **Diamorphine.** Diamorphine consists of two morphine molecules locked together and has a much higher solubility in solution than morphine. Again it is often used epidurally or in continuous infusions.
- **Pethidine.** This drug is prone to accumulation and may lead to serious central nervous system excitement and seizures. Low oral potency and erratic absorption from muscle means it is now rarely used and is particularly unsuitable for the elderly.
- **Methadone.** This synthetic opioid has a long half-life that may be more prolonged in elderly persons.
- **Pentazocine.** This drug is both an agonist and antagonist of opioid receptors and can cause a high incidence of delirium when used in the elderly.
- **Buprenorphene** is also both an agonist and antagonist that can be given sublingually to patients unable to tolerate oral medications. Although there is little published evidence, some elderly patients appear to get on with this drug quite well. Like fentanyl it is now available in patch format for chronic pain management[1].

Local anaesthetics
Nerve blocks are very effective for postoperative pain relief with intercostal nerve blocks aiding pulmonary function after chest or upper abdominal surgery. Pain below the waist can be abolished at rest by an effective continuous epidural infusion. However, blocks spread more widely in the elderly and there may be compromise of respiratory function due to intercostal paralysis. The

[1] Opioid patches should never be used for acute postoperative pain management in any age group.

elderly are also more prone to sympathetic blockade following the administration of epidural or spinal local anaesthetics, resulting in a fall in blood pressure.

Non-pharmacological strategies

Particular attention needs to be paid to comfort. A warm blanket has been found to significantly reduce discomfort, including pain, anxiety and feeling cold (Robinson & Benson 2002). Recovery is likely to be more protracted with patients at greater risk of developing the conditions previously stated, in addition to bed sores and malnutrition. The elderly may not be able to move themselves as easily following surgery and risk lying in one place for too long. Soft mattresses and lifting aids may help to ensure that movement does not lead to further tissue damage during the recovery period.

Distraction can reduce the focus of the pain, so watching the television or listening to the radio or to some pleasant music can be helpful. Gentle massage can be useful too as it stimulates the A-beta fibres (see Chapter 1) and closes the gate, thus reducing input from painful impulses. Sitting with patients for 5–10 minutes and giving them a gentle hand or foot massage is good use of time. Talking, observing and asking about their pain at this time not only allows a skilled assessment but also can be therapeutic in itself.

Resources

- American Society of Anesthesiologists, *Syllabus on Geriatric Anaesthesiology. Post Operative Pain Control in the Elderly Patient* (M.L. Chin): www.asahq.org/clinical/geriatrics/pain_control.htm (accessed October 2005)
- National Institute of Clinical Excellence (NICE) (2001)
- National Prescribing Centre (2002) for additional advice on NSAIDs and specific gastroprotection: *MeReC Briefing* issue no. 20 is available at www.npc.co.uk (accessed October 2005)
- American Medical Association for a very good synopsis on analgesia and adjuvants in the elderly, with specific advice on how these should or should not be used: *Pain Management: Assessing and Treating Pain in Older Adults.* Available at www.ama-cmeonline.com/pain_mgmt/module05/11phar/ (accessed October 2005)
- Ferral & Ferrel (1996), Weiner et al. (2002) and Schofield (2005) for general information on pain in the elderly
- Savage (2005) for information on when Cox-2 inhibitors might be used in the elderly

Trauma

Many elderly people will have evidence of osteoporosis and are therefore at an increased risk of fractures following often quite trivial falls. Even coughing may break a rib in some individuals. Other common fracture sites are hips, wrists and crush fractures of the vertebra.

Experiencing acute trauma pain

> **Case study**
>
> Tom Peters lives alone in a small flat. He was widowed several years ago and apart from occasional breathlessness in the winter or when he has a cold, he declares himself fit and well. He likes to think of himself as 78 years young. He was managing independently, apart from Pat, a local neighbour, who liked to keep an eye out and occasionally did his heavier shopping. Tom was just about to watch TV, when he tripped on a rug, missed grabbing the chair and fell heavily to the floor. The pain in his right leg and hip was excruciating. Unable to move to the telephone he lay overnight willing Pat to call by. Luckily she did but it was 10 a.m. before an ambulance came to take him on the painful journey to hospital. The Accident and Emergency department was busy and he lay on a hard trolley, dreading being moved for the X-ray. He had asked if they could give him something for the pain but the nurses said the doctor was busy with other patients 'if he could just hold on a while'. His mouth felt dry and rough and if it was not for Pat staying with him he could not imagine how he would have coped. She chatted, held his hand and generally fretted about why everything took so long. He just tried to pretend he was not there and as long as he did not move the pain was just bearable.

Pharmacological strategies

In Tom's case, withholding analgesia was inhumane. The introduction of patient group directives for paracetamol and/or an NSAID such as ibuprofen would have enabled rapid intervention with simple analgesia. If either or both of these drugs failed to provide effective analgesia then a low dose of an oral or intravenous opioid such as morphine would be justified. He would quite likely benefit from using an inhalation analgesic such as Entonox for painful positioning for X-rays. Some centres are beginning to offer continuous local anaesthetic blocks to the hip, which may provide very effective analgesia without the side effects of systemic analgesia (Martin & Ali 2002).

Even within a busy Accident and Emergency department, offering a strong opioid and the requirement for close monitoring would not have been an issue as Tom had his friend Pat with him who could have been asked to contact nursing staff if she had any concerns about the quality of Tom's pain control or the level of his sedation. Nurses following specific training can administer intravenous opioids and the use of an algorithm may assist less experienced staff (see Fig. 6.3).

Osteoporosis as a cause of fracture

It is quite possible that Tom's fracture was a result of osteoporosis. In many cases, the pain tends to diminish as the fracture heals; however, vertebral fractures are an exception to this. Whilst some people may be in severe pain that persists long after the fracture has healed, others may not be aware of the injury. Bone normally takes about 3 months to fully heal. Osteoporosis is difficult for many to come to terms with as although it is to some extent treatable, it is an incurable degenerative condition. As with most chronically painful or debilitating diseases, depression can become a factor and treating depression may well help to control pain and improve quality of life.

Pharmacological strategies

For patients suffering from ongoing pain associated with osteoporosis it is important that they and their carers are able to access as much information about effective pharmacological pain management as possible. The following is an example of an advice sheet that a health care professional may go through with a patient. It aims to give as much information as possible about medications so that patients can make more informed choices.

A guideline for managing pain in sufferers of osteoporosis

When pain is difficult to control, taking certain painkillers together is the best approach. Osteoporosis is a chronic condition with no 'cure' so you will need to ensure your pain control is effective and suitable for your needs. The following is a step-by-step guide:

- **Step 1**: for mild pain take 1 g paracetamol (two tablets) four times a day (do not exceed this dose) and try taking it for at least 72 hours so it can reach a steady level in your bloodstream. Remember to take paracetamol regularly. Just taking one or two tablets when pain becomes intolerable may not give a true picture of how effective this painkiller can be. Paracetamol is safe and can be taken by the very young and the very old as long as the normal dose is not exceeded, which for adults is eight tablets per day.
- **Step 2**: for pain that is not getting better following step 1, add in 400 mg ibuprofen (an anti-inflammatory drug) three times a day with meals. Some patients may need to take additional medicine to protect their stomachs. Elderly patients or those with a previous history of gastric ulcer, indigestion, heart or kidney disease or with a blood clotting disorder may have to avoid anti-inflammatory medicines altogether. If you suffer with asthma made worse by aspirin or ibuprofen you will also need an alternative painkiller. Discuss with your doctor or pharmacist any concerns you may have.
- **Step 3**: if your pain relief is still not particularly effective it may be worth stopping ibuprofen and replacing it with a different anti-inflammatory pain killer that works in the same way, such as 150 mg diclofenac in 24 hours. This is only available on prescription. Anti-inflammatory medicines must not be taken if you are prescribed warfarin and should not be used for long periods of time. Try to reduce all doses after 5 days' continuous use.

    Although these medicines can be very effective, many patients cannot tolerate them or the newer ones called Cox-2 drugs. However, getting on top of pain quickly before it can become established using a combination of drugs and therapies is effective. An ibuprofen or diclofenac cream may be an alternative if you cannot take the tablets.

- **Step 4**: If pain is still not well controlled on the combination of a full dose of paracetamol and an anti-inflammatory medication, ask your doctor if you can try including a low dose of a strong painkiller. In the past codeine or dihydrocodeine were added at this stage. If they are effective then they can be continued. However, we now know that codeine and dihydrocodeine are not usually effective painkillers on their own and they can cause nausea, sedation, unsteadiness and constipation for little additional benefit once steps 1, 2 or 3 have failed. You may obtain improved pain control by trying oral morphine.

How to take strong painkillers

If codeine is prescribed, you should feel some benefit after the first or second full dose (60 mg codeine or 30 mg dihydrocodeine). Writing down in a diary if your painkiller has had any effect is a good way of deciding whether to continue with it or not. Make a note of how bad your pain is before taking a dose (this can usually be done using a scale of 0—10, with 0 = no pain and 10 = worst pain ever, or using a verbal scale such as none, mild, moderate, severe or excruciating pain). After a couple of hours make a note again of how bad your pain is and how much, if any, the painkiller was able to reduce it. If your pain control is not improved then these drugs can be confidently discontinued. Codeine and dihydrocodeine work by being converted in your body to morphine and some people are unable to do this, so it is important not to take these drugs if they are not working for you.

If an episode of severe pain requires a stronger painkiller, then the most appropriate in the short term may be oral morphine syrup (2 mg/ml). The effective dose range is usually 5—20 mg (half to two teaspoons) repeated four to six times a day. It is only possible to establish the effective dose for you by starting low and gradually increasing the dose. Be sure to keep a record of any improvements in your pain control but also if you experience side effects such as drowsiness or nausea. If you are drowsy this is a sign that the last dose of morphine you had was too large. You can reduce your next dose, leave a longer gap between doses or omit the next dose altogether. You will not be able to drive or operate any machinery after taking oral morphine and for at least 7 hours after your last dose.

If your pain is lasting for weeks or months rather than days but morphine is still helpful, a long-acting tablet will tend to cause fewer side effects with more consistent pain control and will be easier to use. This will need to be reviewed regularly with your doctor and the dose gradually reduced when pain eventually subsides.

A preparation such as oxycodone (10 mg extended release morning and evening) may reduce sedation, nausea and hallucinations if you experience these side effects with morphine. If tablets or syrup prove unsuitable for you your doctor may prescribe a 'patch' releasing a strong painkiller over 72 hours.

All these drugs cause constipation, but this can usually be treated by increasing your fluid and roughage intake and by taking a laxative as needed.

Many patients and health care professions fear the risk of addiction. This is highly unlikely to occur whilst strong painkillers are being taken for short periods of time to control initial pain.

Further guidance on taking these medicines is available from the British Pain Society, which has produced an excellent booklet for patients, via www.britishpainsociety.org.

The key to safe use of all painkillers is to take them as soon as pain becomes problematic and for short periods only (i.e. a few days or weeks). Pain once it is out of control is always harder to treat. Stop any painkillers that are not relieving your pain. Some sorts of pain cannot be controlled by any of the traditional painkillers and you may need other forms of treatment or a specialist referral.

Other medication treatments

Treating the problem is important in order to reduce further bone damage and there are medicines that help with this. Calcitonin is a natural substance produced by the body that may slow the loss of bone and relieve pain associated with fractures. Calcium and vitamin D are important to bone health but need to be taken following advice. If pain is causing your sleep to be disturbed,

5–25 mg amitriptyline taken at night may be effective. This medication is useful for certain types of pain. Although it is an antidepressant it is prescribed to treat your pain and not because your doctor thinks you are depressed. The pain may make you feel low in mood, but the 'antidepressant' acts centrally to alleviate pain in ways that are not always clearly understood.

Non-pharmacological strategies
Reducing the number of painkillers you take may be important if you are taking other non-painkilling medications. Taking painkillers and using non-drug therapies together can help you to achieve this.

- **Heat and cold**: warm showers or hot packs can help to relieve pain or stiff muscles and can add to feelings of comfort. Cold applied for no more than 15–20 minutes at a time also helps reduce swelling and inflammation. Always place a towel between your skin and the source of cold or heat to protect your skin.
- **Braces and supports**: these are sometimes used following a fracture in your back.
- **Exercise**: this is needed to prevent your muscles from weakening and to increase your strength and balance. A regular but gentle exercise programme started as soon as possible can also improve your energy and help you to remain independent.
- **Acupuncture and acupressure**: these may be useful for some people.
- **Massage therapy**: massage can help to relax stiff muscles and increase blood supply. If you have osteoporosis in your back, it must be gentle and not done near your spine.
- **Relaxation**: this involves concentration and slow, deep breathing to release tension from muscles. It requires some training to do effectively. Music may help you concentrate on this technique.
- **Distraction**: when pain is particularly troublesome try to focus on pictures of pleasant scenes, events and happy memories or watch your favourite television programme as this may help you to feel less pain.

CHRONIC PAIN

For the elderly, in addition to the neuropathic and muscoloskeletal pains mentioned in Chapter 6, there is an increased risk of patients becoming affected by rheumatoid arthritis (RA) and/or osteoarthritis (OA) (Ferrell & Ferrell 1996; Jakobsson & Hallberg 2002). Although RA and OA may commonly start around the age of 40, by the age of 75 at least 85% of the population have either clinical and/or radiological evidence of OA (Davis 1988; Sack 1995). Other common sources of chronic pain in the elderly include heart disease and angina, metabolic disorders such as diabetes, neurological conditions such as Parkinson's, cancer and general aches and pain associated with reduced mobility, decreasing function and associated impairment.

Principles of assessment and evaluation for chronic pain

The assessment of chronic pain is essential for the development and evaluation of an individual plan of care specific to an elderly patient's needs and concurrent therapy. The assessment of acute pain can be relatively quick and tools are frequently simple scales, whereas chronic pain assessment needs to reflect the multidimensional nature of pain and the tools include more than just the 'intensity' of the pain. The elderly especially may need additional help to be able to understand and contribute to the assessment process. It is not unusual for other 'assessments' to be included, such as 'quality of life' (QoL) and mobility, which again can be an important factor for elderly patients. Patience is needed to ask questions and wait for responses. Chronic pain can permeate many facets of life and it is important to include a general

---

Box 7.5 Managing pain in the community setting

Older People – Managing Their Pain in the Community Setting (Schofield et al. 2005) is a wonderful resource available on the Internet and is organised as a case study. You take the role of a community nurse visiting an elderly lady who has considerable pain, diabetes and osteoporosis. As well as giving extensive detail, questions are asked throughout and some very good answers and references are provided.

Box 7.6 Pain in the cognitively impaired patient

According to Ferrell et al. (1995) pain reports from older people with cognitive impairment were as reliable and valid as people without impairment. Pain was assessed using the McGill pain questionnaire and four unidimensional scales previously used with younger adults. Eighty three percent were capable of completing at least one unidimensional pain assessment scale. Those who were not able to complete the scale could identify the pain in response to a direct question.

---

question about how pain might also affect sleep, appetite, mood, function and social activity (see Box 7.5). It is important to include multidimensional tools as sleep and function are good indicators of pain. The essence of sound assessment should include (Hanks-Bell et al. 2004) the following:

- Quality of the pain
- Location
- Intensity
- Onset pattern and duration
- Exacerbating and alleviating features
- Response to previous treatments

It is not inevitable that older people will experience cognitive impairment, but sadly for many it is a fact of life. For these individuals, pain assessment can be particularly challenging (see Box 7.6).

Short form McGill Pain Questionnaire (SF-MPQ) (see Fig. 6.7)
This tool may not be suitable for the elderly if cognitive impairment or concentration are issues. Even in its short form it will take several minutes to complete.

Brief Pain Inventory (see Fig. 1.6)
Again this may be complicated for some elderly to complete but can be useful if patients are assisted by staff. The data will provide a good base line on which pain management strategies can be assessed as they are introduced.

Assessing pain in patients with cognitive impairment
The following are some of the specific assessment tools either in use or under development for assessing pain in cognitively impaired patients.

The Assessment of Discomfort in Dementia (ADD) protocol
The ADD protocol is a systematic tool that can be used by nurses to make a differential assessment and treatment plan for both physical pain and affective discomfort experienced by people with dementia. The ADD protocol is based on the assumption that behaviours associated with dementia are symptoms of unmet physiological and/or non-physiological needs. See Kovach et al. (2002).

Checklist of Non-verbal Pain Indicators (CNPI)
This instrument was designed to measure pain behaviour in cognitively impaired older people. Instrument testing was conducted on a population of elderly patients with hip fractures. Inter-rater reliability is the extent to which 'raters' (who administer the interview/questionnaire, etc.) get the same results. In other words, how consistent they are or well trained. The reliability showed 93% agreement on the dichotomous checklist items. Behaviours occurred more frequently during movement in this population. Of the six pain-related behaviours in the instrument, facial grimaces/winces occurred in 44% of the patients tested. Observed pain behaviours were positively correlated with self-reports of pain. See Feldt (2000).

Discomfort Scale-dementia of the Alzheimer's Type (DS-DAT)
This is an established research tool for assessing discomfort in patients with dementia. It does not have comprehensive pain-

related indicators and is less used in clinical practice. See Hurley et al. (1992).

DOLOPLUS 2

DOLOPLUS 2 is used to assess pain in the elderly with dementia based upon clinicians' observations of patient behaviour in ten different situations, such as somatic complaint, washing/dressing, mobility, communication, social life and problems of behaviour. See Lefebvre-Chapiro et al. (2001).

Nursing Assistant-administered Instrument to Assess Pain in Demented Individuals (NOPPAIN)

NOPPAIN was designed for use by nursing assistants to assess the pain of nursing-home residents with dementia. The presence and intensity of six pain behaviours (pain words, pain faces, pain noises, bracing, rubbing, restlessness) are assessed. Simple wording and icons minimise the English reading level required. See Snow et al. (2004).

Pain Assessment Scale for Seniors with Severe Dementia (PACSLAC)

PACSLAC is for use with patients with severe dementia. The tool has four subsets and although it has a total of 60 items, it is reported to be easy and not time consuming to use. See Fuchs-Lacelle and Hadjistavropoulos (2004).

Pain Assessment for the Dementing Elderly (PADE)

Again for use with severe dementia, PADE has three parts with a total of 24 items but is reported to take just 5–10 minutes to complete. See Villanueva et al. (2003).

Pain Assessment in Advanced Dementia (PAINAD) scale

A third tool for assessing pain in patients with severe dementia is that of the PAINAD scale. See Warden et al. (2003).

Pain Assessment Tool in Confused Older Adults (PATCOA)

PATCOA is another tool for use with confused older adults. It was initially evaluated with cognitively intact older patients undergoing orthopaedic surgery. See Decker and Perry (2003).

Chronic musculoskeletal pain

Rheumatoid arthritis (RA)
(See also the section on juvenile rheumatoid arthritis in Chapter 5.)

Case study

Pamela is 60 years old and has managed to cope with her rheumatoid arthritis since first diagnosed with the condition 20 years ago, using just herbal remedies and supplements. Her mother also had the condition and as Pamela knew what it was, she never sought help from her doctor or considered any medical intervention until now as the joints in her hand have become increasing inflamed and painful. The pain is interfering with her daily life.

Rheumatoid arthritis is a chronic systemic condition involving inflammation of peripheral joints, resulting in progressive destruction of the joint's articular and periarticular structure. Its incidence increases up to the age of 80 and it is a major cause of disability and pain in the elderly. There is some speculation that late onset RA may be a different condition to that experienced in younger people (Kavanaugh 1997). However, its cause is still unknown, although research is continuing to improve understanding.

Rheumatic diseases are sometimes classified as follows:

- Immune-based joint diseases such rheumatoid arthritis and ankylosing spondylitis
- Connective tissue diseases such as systemic lupus erythematosis and scleroderma
- Infectious arthritis
- Crystal deposit diseases such as gout
- Soft tissue rheumatism such as tendinitis and bursitis
- Bone disorders such as osteoporosis and Paget's disease

In rheumatoid arthritis, synovial tissue becomes hyperplastic, infiltrated with lymphocytes and plasma cells, whilst inflammatory substances such as cytokines, prostaglandins and immunoglobulins are released in the synovial fluid. The disease may attack primarily the joints of the hands and feet, but larger joints such as elbows, shoulders and knees may also be affected. Pain can be severe with swelling and stiffness especially in the morning. It is a distressing feature that leads to loss of function. Extra-articular features are also common and may involve multiple organ systems (Lee & Weinblatt 2001).

This systemic disease process may shorten life, with a higher risk of serious infection or the development of cardiovascular disease. Treatment is based on disease modification and symptom control. It should be multimodal and subjected to regular review. Therefore treatment is usually superior when undertaken by a team of rheumatological specialists. Co-morbidity and polypharmacy can complicate the care of the elderly, making their symptom control very challenging.

Pharmacological strategies

NSAIDs and Cox-2 inhibitors
These drugs have been the mainstay of pain control in RA sufferers using regular full doses and often over the long term to inhibit prostaglandin synthesis. However, the problems associated with these drugs are considerably increased in elderly RA sufferers. As discussed previously, these analgesics need careful selection and monitoring in the older person and updated information should be consulted from reputable sources such as Bandolier, the National Institute for Health and Clinical Excellence (NICE) and the Food and Drug Administration (FDA).

Opioids
Currently opioids do not appear to be routinely used in rheumatoid arthritis but may well provide analgesia, if the pain is resistant to other treatments, in much the same way as opioids are used to control the initial pain of osteoporosis. The development of novel opioids that act outside the central nervous system may offer some benefit in the future (Walker 2001). Work has also been conducted on intra-articular opioid receptors, codeine and tramadol (Budd 1994; Konttinen et al. 1994). Low doses of strong opioids are possibly less constipating than large doses of weak

ones, with preparations such as buprenorphine or fentanyl in a patch format seemingly causing the least constipation. Patches may well be more effective when forgetfulness, poor compliance, concordance or problems with renal function make using regular oral opioids problematic for pain that has been established as 'opioid responsive'. Unfortunately there are very little data published on this so far and many texts continue to advocate the use of weak opioids such as codeine and dihydrocodeine. One recent study has shown that excellent results can be obtained using strong opioids, but more research is needed and hopefully this will be more forthcoming in the future (Walker 2001).

Corticosteroids
Corticosteroids can improve pain and symptom control, but long term their use is associated with osteoporosis, cataracts, poor wound healing, hyperglycaemia, hypertension, hyperlipidaemia and an increased risk of infection. To minimise these risks the drugs can also be given intra-articularly to control symptoms when only one or two joints are affected.

Disease-modifying anti-rheumatic drugs (DMARDs)
DMARDs are given to reduce symptoms by slowing down the disease process. There is little evidence that the elderly are at greater risk using these drugs, especially methotrexate, providing they are monitored closely. Routine determination of serum liver enzymes and renal function may reduce individual risk (Hirshberg et al. 2000).

Capsaicin cream
This may help by reducing the influence of substance P (Konttinen et al. 1994).

Gold injections
Gold injections are also thought to affect substance P production (Konttinen et al. 1994).

Tricyclic antidepressants
These drugs can be very problematic in the elderly due to their adverse side effect profile, but they may improve sleep and act

on descending modulation via the noradrenalin and seratonin inhibition pathway (Konttinen et al. 1994; Shipton 1999). A randomised clinical trial (RCT) study of female patients with RA and depression/anxiety reported that dothiepin relieved pain and disability (Ash et al. 1999), but more data are required. Surgery is an option when other treatment has failed and there is joint destruction.

Non-pharmacological strategies

Physical activity
Keeping active seems to be vital to maintaining function and improving pain control (Stenstrom 1994). Devices may assist in encouraging interesting activities such as gardening. Patients may also need some assistance, including aids and devices to help them get dressed and with eating, etc.

Older adults with chronic illnesses or disabilities can gain significant health benefits with a moderate amount of physical activity, especially if this is done daily. A recent review of individually tailored programmes for elderly people demonstrated that programmes to build muscle strength, improve balance and promote walking significantly reduced falls in older persons (Gillespie et al. 2002). Gentle exercise may help individials cope with chronic pain.

Promoting physical activity in older adults depends on the following:

- Assess how much physical activity patients are enjoying and explore reasons why they are not more active.
- Substantial health benefits occur with a moderate amount of activity (e.g. at least 30 minutes of brisk walking) on five or more days of the week.
- Brief episodes of physical activity, as little as 10 minutes at a time, can be beneficial if repeated. Sedentary patients can begin with brief episodes and gradually increase the duration or intensity of activity.
- Moderate amounts of low-impact activities such as swimming, water exercises or stretching are recommended for those who have difficulty with their mobility.

- Refer patients to community resources where they can join group activities to promote and reinforce physical activity.

Just as for acute pain, distraction therapy and relaxation techniques may also prove very beneficial.

Rest
This of course may be needed when symptoms are very severe, but prolonged bed rest in the elderly can rapidly lead to further disability and advice to rest has been largely based on little evidence (Kidd 2002). Restoration of function must be the goal to ensure that the elderly can retain some mobility despite their pain and handicap.

TENS
Some benefit is possibly provided by TENS in rheumatological conditions (Konttinen et al. 1994; Nicholas 1994). The elderly will often experience considerable difficulty siting the pads as flexibility declines with age.

Coping and behavioural therapy
Positive coping strategies need to be reinforced. Passive avoidance, catastrophising, an external locus of control, hoping it will get better on its own and depression are all poor psychological indicators for improvement or maintaining a reasonable quality of life (Lambert et al. 1990). An internal locus of control, active information seeking and cognitive restructuring can help patients to adapt and cope better with their disease, helping them to remain active and engaged with life (Kitte 1966). The best predictor of psychological well-being appears to be the emotion of challenge, optimism and self-reliance (Downe-Wamboldt & Melanson 1998).

The following non-pharmacological therapies are often included in articles and advice sheets to patients, but the evidence to support them is not robust. As with many complementary therapies, research methodology may be a factor leading to weak conclusions (see Box 7.7). However, many patients do report positive effects.

Box 7.7 Systematic reviews (Moore et al. 2003)

Systematic reviews have not been able to conclude that homeopathy, relaxation or acupuncture reduce pain in older people. There is some support for:

- The herb 'feverfew' to prevent migraines
- Quinine to reduce leg cramps
- Vegetarian diets being beneficial for rheumatoid arthritis

- An individual exercise regime, movement and posture re-education
- Deep breathing
- Cold and heat applied both for pain relief and to help reduce stiffness in joints
- Massage
- Meditation and guided imagery
- Therapeutic touch
- Chiropractic treatment
- Acupuncture and acupressure
- Magnet therapy
- Herb treatments
- Shark cartilage
- Vitamin supplements
- Mineral supplements such as zinc, copper, selenium, manganese
- Bee pollen, royal jelly and evening primrose

Resources

- Belostocki & Paget (2002)
- Merck (2005)
- Bandolier: www.jr2.ox.ac.uk/bandolier (accessed October 2005)
- Prodigy (2005)
- National Guideline Clearinghouse (2004)
- Arthritis Care: www.arthritiscare.org.uk/home/index.cfm?region=uk (accessed October 2005)
- National Rheumatoid Arthritis Society, a patient support group that is part of the British Society for Rheumatology: www.rheumatology.org.uk/link/patient_support_links/rheumatoid (accessed October 2005)
- Dessein et al. (2000) for further information on rheumatological pain

> **Box 7.8 Pain and quality of life in older people with arthritis**
>
> A literature review by Jakobsson & Hallberg (2002) exploring pain and quality of life (QoL) in older people with rheumatoid arthritis and/or osteoarthritis found that increased age did relate to pain and a decrease in QoL. Whilst there were insufficient studies on people over 75 years of age the authors concluded that these people should be assessed for their levels of pain, functional limitations and QoL. Social networks/support appeared to have a major impact on people's lives and might be the reason why some people with a good social network 'cope' with pain better than those with less social support.

Osteoarthritis

> **Case study**
>
> Brian is a 71 year old gentleman who is becoming increasing debilitated with arthritis in both hips. He finds walking very difficult, which is having a substantial impact on his quality of life. The analgesics he was taking have become less effective but he has been reluctant to consider surgery at his age. He rarely sleeps for more than two hours at any one time and is becoming very despondent and fatigued.

Osteoarthritis is a common joint disease, with knees and hips the most commonly affected joints. The condition affects around 10–20% of over 65 year olds. It is regarded as a degenerative disease presenting with roughened cartilage that becomes thin whilst the bone underneath thickens. Osteophytes or bony spurs may develop as the thickened bone at the edge of the joints grows outwards. The joint may swell, ligaments contract and muscles weaken and waste. Stiff and painful joints are a feature, but the disease is unrelated to rheumatoid arthritis. Symptoms may resolve spontaneously for weeks or months at a time. Pain of this type can severely impact on the quality of life for these people (see Box 7.8).

Pharmacological strategies
Simple analgesia such as 1 g paracetamol regularly for acute flares is the mainstay; however, remaining on any drugs for a long period of time cannot be recommended. Combined painkillers

(the 'Co' drugs) are still used extensively in the elderly with OA but bring all the problems associated with codeine and the weak opioids mentioned previously. Tramadol may have a place as a weak opioid, but it also acts on the pain-modulating pathways associated with seratonin and noradrenalin and therefore may offer some benefit (Rosenthal et al. 2004). Nefopam and meptazinol are sometimes suggested as alternatives to morphine or similar opioids. The place for strong opioids has yet to be fully established, but when pain is limiting mobilisation, a monitored and sensible regime that may include oral strong opioids for pain unresponsive to other treatments may improve quality of life and mobility for the older person.

If inflammation of the joint is present NSAIDs may also have a place, but their side effect profile in the elderly means they must be used with caution and probably only for a very limited period in OA (Visser et al. 2002). If pain is confined to just one or two joint areas then topical NSAID that does not have the adverse side effect profile may provide sufficient analgesia.

Capsaicin cream is safe and can be effective for some individuals who can tolerate the burning sensation on application. Steroid injections can also provide symptom relief, especially when combined with an increase in mobility (Dessein et al. 1999).

Non-pharmacological strategies

Heat and cool
Heat and cool can be soothing but will not alter the course of the disease.

Weight and obesity
Patients who are overweight should be advised to reduce their weight in order to minimise stress on joints. Interestingly, obesity is actually a risk factor for osteoarthritis due to increased mechanical stress on the cartilage.

Music
Music has been shown to elevate mood and increase feelings of control in older people. A study by McCaffery & Freeman (2003) using a randomised controlled trial examined the influence of

music on older people with osteoarthritis ($n = 66$). Those who listened to music had less pain compared to those who did not. They concluded that listening to music for 20 minutes each day was effective in reducing pain for older people living in the community.

Exercise
This will help with weight control but will also help to keep joints functioning and maintain blood supply to the tissues. Strengthening exercises are designed to improve strength and muscle tone, thus stabilising joints. These exercises are particularly important in the elderly as they can reduce the risk of falls. Aerobic exercise can help to reduce pain and improve sleep and well-being. Although pain initially may limit mobilisation, exercise is vital and patients should be encouraged to take pre-emptive analgesics and continue with the regime for several weeks to gain maximum benefit. The elderly may find exercise difficult to achieve because of problems getting to see a physiotherapist, and costs associated with travel, obtaining self-help books or videos may well be significant issues on a pension. The elderly are not usually associated with vigorous use of the Internet in order to download information either but a relative may be able to help, especially an enthusiastic grandchild!

Pacing activity levels
Being able to pace activity means spreading chores through the day rather than getting into a pattern of overdoing things when pain is bearable and then suffering later and spending too much time inactive whilst trying to recover.

Shoes
These need to be relatively flat and have a thick rubber sole to act as a shock absorber.

A walking stick
This may help to take some of the pressure off a painful joint but will need to be matched to a patient's height and advice should be given to ensure it is used correctly (Schwameder et al. 1999).

TENS
TENS has been reported as beneficial in rheumatological conditions and may be useful in other forms of joint pain (Nicholas 1994). Again, TENS may be a struggle for the elderly to apply and there are the cost implications to consider also.

Glucosamine and chondroitin tablets
Although these remain popular, research is currently trying to establish benefit, but many patients appear to do well when these supplements are taken for several months.

Surgery
This can offer a solution when all else has failed, with joint replacements becoming more and more sophisticated.

Resources
- Arthritis Care:18 Stephenson Way, London, NW1 2HD. Telephone helpline: 0808 800 4050. See www.arthritiscare.org.uk (accessed October 2005)
- The Arthritis Foundation, an American organisation: www.arthritis.org/conditions/diseasecenter/oa.asp (accessed October 2005)

Neuropathic pain

Case study

Margaret is a 92 year old lady suffering from severe trigeminal neuralgia. She has had this condition for many years and it has been adequately controlled with carbamazepine. However, her admission to hospital was brought about because she suddenly became very ill, was falling over and becoming increasingly confused. A urinary tract infection was diagnosed, but the levels of carbamazepine in her blood suggested toxicity. The carbamazepine was discontinued. Although Mary's other conditions had stabilised her facial pain was intolerable. She could not eat properly and even speaking was becoming increasingly painful. The pain team were called.

Pharmacological strategies

A trial of gapapentin was instigated. Even at top dose this was not sufficient to control Margaret's pain to the level she had obtained on carbamazepine. Eventually pain control was re-established with a low dose of carbamazepine in addition to a moderate dose of gapapentin. Mary was intolerant to even low doses of a range of tricyclic antidepressants.

Usually carbamazepine is first-line treatment for this pain, which does not respond to simple analgesia. Other medications include gabapentin, phenytoin, baclofen, lamotrigine, valproic acid and clonazepam, which have all been reviewed by McQuay et al. (1995).

Opioids are not usually used for this condition, but this may not necessarily be because they are ineffective and may simply reflect long-held beliefs and prejudice. However, as the main side effect of the most effective pharmacological therapy carbamazepin is central nervous system depression, attempting to trial a strong opioid in addition often proves intolerable for the patient.

Non-pharmacological strategies

Surgical options
The pathology of trigeminal neuralia is thought to involve neurovascular compression of the trigeminal nerve as it leaves the brain stem. Microvascular decompression surgery is now well established. Rhizotomy using radiofrequency or glycerol and nerve compression using a balloon may also provide some pain relief (Taha & Twe 1996).

Acupuncture
This is sometimes cited as a treatment but there is a lack of research in this area. Some people do experience positive effects though and should not be discouraged from having acupuncture if this is the case.

Biofeedback
Biofeedback has been suggested, but the usefulness of this strategy may be limited in some elderly. However, Gagliese &

Melzack (1997) undertook a review of the treatment of chronic pain in the elderly and suggested that reductions in pain intensity and medication intake may be achieved when training for using biofeedback and relaxation techniques were simplified.

Resources

- Prodigy guidelines: www.prodigy.nhs.uk/guidance.asp?gt=trigeminal%20 neuralgia (accessed October 2005)
- Trigeminal Neuralgia Association UK: an American organisation but with lots of useful information; see www.tna-support.org. Also their patient support home site: www.tna.org.uk/index.php (both accessed October 2005)
- National Institute of Neurological Disorders and Stroke: again an American organisation and website but it has useful links; see www.ninds.nih.gov/ disorders/trigeminal_neuralgia/trigeminal_neuralgia.htm (accessed October 2005)

Chronic visceral pain

Case study

Robert is a 78 year old gentleman who has been diagnosed by his general practitioner with stable angina. He has been prescribed drugs specifically to help control the painful symptoms of this condition. Invasive investigations and possibly surgery have been discussed with Robert but he is very reluctant to consider going down this route. He has come to see you, at the nurse practitioner clinic, for advice about how and when to take medication to control his pain and to discuss lifestyle changes that may be beneficial in reducing the impact of his condition

Stable angina is characterised by chest pain and discomfort on exertion, particularly walking up a hill, following meals or during emotional stress. The pain may typically radiate to the neck, jaw, back and sometimes the arms. Patients will sometimes recount feelings of fear, dread, choking, squeezing and crushing, making the whole experience very unpleasant. With stable angina symptoms can usually be relieved by rest and/or anti-angina medications. As this pain comes from a blockage in the coronary arteries simply taking a painkiller would not be effective. Conservative treatment of the condition centres on controlling the symptoms in order to provide pain relief.

Pharmacological strategies
Nitrates are usually the first-line therapy for angina pain and are available in various preparations, including fast-acting sublingual nitroglycerin to provide immediate relief. To reduce the frequency of angina attacks drugs to control hypercholesterolaemia and aspirin for its antiplatelet activity are usually given. Beta-blockers are widely used but can be associated with side effects such as depression, which can impact on pain-coping strategies. Calcium channel blockers are also effective but are currently under scrutiny for potentially increasing the risk of mortality in certain patients.

Non-pharmacological strategies

Weight and obesity
If overweight, patients should be encouraged to reduce to as close to their optimum weight as possible. This may not be easy as many elderly live alone and taking care to prepare nutritious meals, which are high in fibre and low in salt, may be seen as an unwanted chore and shopping regularly for fresh ingredients may be problematic. Bad eating habits can be very hard to break and if patients feel depressed then food can become a comfort strategy.

Exercise
Exercise should be taken regularly and built up gradually to increase exercise tolerance. Exercise can help with weight loss and improve general feelings of well-being. For many elderly people, they will only be successful if taking part in some group exercise therapy with other individuals suffering from heart disease. It is important they have some professional input to ensure they are exercising correctly and within their capabilities.

Stress
Stress when it is prolonged and potentially damaging should be avoided if possible, although a little excitement may be beneficial!

Relaxation techniques

Along with group exercise, relaxation techniques often have to be learnt. Unless patients can participate in rehabilitation classes the elderly especially may struggle to develop worthwhile techniques. Videos, books and pamphlets are important sources of information but rely on good eyesight or an ability to use a machine such as a video recorder or DVD player.

Alcohol

Some people find that alcohol helps them to relax, but this should be limited to no more than the recommended units per week.

Surgery

Surgery is also an option for this condition and is being undertaken successfully on patients of increasing age. The techniques include percutaneous transluminal coronary angioplasty (PTCA), which involves heart catheterisation to guide a balloon to dilate a blocked coronary artery. Other alternatives are atherectomy, stent placement or a coronary artery bypass graft (CABG).

Resources

- National Guideline Clearinghouse: www.guideline.gov (accessed October 2005)
- Scottish Intercollegiate Guidelines Network (SIGN): www.sign.ac.uk/index.html (accessed October 2005)
- BUPA health fact sheet: www.hcd2.bupa.co.uk/fact_sheets/html/angina.html (accessed October 2005)
- British Heart Foundation: tel. 020 7935 0185, www.bhf.org.uk (accessed October 2005)

Overcoming potential barriers specific to the elderly

Several barriers, patient and professional, have been identified that affect older people and the management of their chronic pain. As mentioned in the assessment section, changes such as sensory or cognitive impairment can make assessment difficult. Some of these challenges can be overcome by using assessment tools that have been specifically developed to address the issue of cognitive impairment. However, the following strategies may also help overcome some of these barriers:

- Identify any sensory loss (e.g. impaired hearing or vision) and ensure that patients have their hearing appliance in place or their glasses are available and clean.
- If language is a barrier then perhaps a relative could act as a translator. Otherwise some larger hospitals or community services (Citizens Advice Bureau) will often have a list of people who could provide this service.
- Communicate clearly and position yourself close to patients, allowing them to see you. Sometimes if they can do this they will be able to read your lips. Avoid standing at the end of the bed or across the room. Try not to raise your voice.
- Use touch to convey your interest in their pain – gentle physical contact on the back of the hand or forearm can convey a great deal and enhances active listening.
- Explore the older persons' personal beliefs about their pain. They might believe it is inevitable with age or they do not want to be a burden.
- Include the family or carer where possible as they may be able to give valuable additional information.
- Always select an appropriate pain assessment tool and document the assessment on a regular basis.

It has been noted that professionals may inadvertently have misconceptions about older people and pain, such as fears about drug toxicity and addiction (McCaffery & Beebe 1994). A survey of 121 nursing homes in the north of England found that 40% of qualified staff and 85% of care assistants had no specialist knowledge regarding the management of pain in older people (Allcock et al. 2002). This has significant implications for the effective management of pain in older people in residential care.

Cognitive impairment can mask the expression of pain. Research has shown that severely demented patients are at risk of underdetection and undertreatment of their pain (Morrison 2000). Deterioration of one or more of the following can indicate cognitive impairment (Ferrell 1996):

- Memory – not being able to recall recent events
- Attention – difficulty listening or watching TV for concentrated periods of time

- Visual spatial skills – difficulty picking up an object or judging distances
- Language – difficulty finding the words to express thoughts or feelings
- Behaviour – changes in normal behaviour

Although few studies have addressed the value of the family in pain assessment, it would appear that family members can be particularly good at recognising when an older relative has pain (SUPPORT Investigators 1995). The accuracy of family members reporting patients' pain has been found to be correct up to 80% of the time and when patients denied pain nearly 70% of the time (Desbiens & Mueller-Rizner 2000; Desbiens & Wu 2000). Because the family can offer such a valuable contribution they should be included where possible in any education sessions so they too may become familiar with pain assessment tools. Whenever pain is suspected a documented pain assessment completed before a therapeutic trial of an analgesic may help to build the effectiveness profile of interventions.

SUMMARY

To summarise, in the elderly it is preferable to use two or three interventions, such as analgesics with non-pharmacological strategies. Interviews with 90 older people receiving home care in Sweden, who were experiencing persistent pain, revealed that the most common strategies used were: medication, rest, mobility, distracting activities and talking about pain (Blomqvist & Edberg 2002). The elderly can have considerable co-morbidity and may be taking multiple medications that may interact. Analgesic doses often have to be reduced and particular care taken with evaluation. Paracetamol is considered the safest drug in the elderly but can be toxic to the liver at a dose of above 4 g in 24 hours. NSAIDs must be used with great caution as they are associated with a high risk of adverse events especially in the elderly (see Bandolier, NSAIDs and Adverse Effects, www.jr2.ox.ac.uk/bandolier/booth/painpag/nsae/nsae.html). Measurable pharmacokinetic changes result in higher, more prolonged plasma drug concentrations, which increase the risk of toxicity and adverse side effects.

We know that the consequences of unrelieved pain in the older person have a significant impact on their physical and psychological well-being. All too often pain is accepted as an inevitable part of getting older. This chapter has demonstrated that older people have specific considerations regarding their pain but successful management is possible, especially when a careful assessment precedes the use of pharmacological and non–pharmacological interventions.

REFERENCES

Abbey, J., Piller, N., De Bellis, A., et al. (2004) The Abbey pain scale: a 1-minute numerical indicator for people with end-stage dementia. *International Journal of Palliative Nursing* **10** (1), 6–13.

Acute Pain Management Guidelines Panel (1992) *Acute Pain Management: Operative or Medical Procedures and Trauma: Clinical Practice Guidelines*. AHCPR Publ. no. 92–0032. Agency for Health Care Policy and Research, Public Health Service, US Department of Health and Human Services, Rockville, Maryland.

Allcock, N., McGarry, J. & Elkan, R. (2002) Management of pain in older people within the nursing home: a preliminary study. *Health and Social Care in the Community* **10** (6), 464–471.

American Medical Association (2005) *Featured CSA Report: Improving the Quality of Geriatric Pharmacotherapy*. Available at www.ama-assn.org/ama/pub/category/13592.html#pharmcoepidemiology, accessed October 2005.

Ash, G., Dickens, C., Creed, F., Jayson, M. & Tomenson, B. (1999) The effects of dothiepin on subjects with rheumatoid arthritis and depression. *Rheumatology* **38** (10), 959–967.

Aubrun, F., Monsel, S., Langeron, O., Coriat, P. & Riou, B. (2002) Post-operative titration of intravenous morphine in the elderly patient. *Anesthesiology* **96** (1),17–23.

Bandolier (2005) *Cox-2 Roundup*. Available at www.jr2.ox.ac.uk/bandolier/band75/b75-2.html. accessed October 2005.

Bannwarth, B., Fabienne Pehourcq, F., Lagrange, F., et al. (2001) Single and multiple dose pharmacokinetics of acetaminophen (paracetamol) in polymedicated very old patients with rheumatic pain. *Journal of Rheumatology* **28** (1), 182–184.

Belostocki, K. & Paget, S.(2002) *Postgraduate Medicine. Inflammatory Rheumatologic Disorders in the Elderly. Unusual Presentations, Altered Outlooks*. Available at www.postgradmed.com/issues/2002/04_02/belostocki1.htm, accessed October 2005.

Bird, J. (2005) Assessing pain in older people. *Nursing Standard* **19** (19), 45–54.

Blomqvist, K. (2003) Older people in persistent pain: nurse and para-medical staff perceptions and pain management. *Journal of Advanced Nursing* **41** (6), 575–584.

Blomqvist, K. & Edberg, A.K. (2002) Living with persistent pain: experiences of older people receiving home care. *Journal of Advanced Nursing* **40** (3), 297–306.

Blower, A.L., Brooks, A., Fenn, G.C., et al. (1997) Emergency admissions for upper GI disease and their relation to NSAID use. *Ailmentary Pharmacology and Therapeutics* **11**, 283–291.

Bombardier, C., Laine, L., Reicin, A., et al., for the VIGOR Study Group (2001) Comparison of upper gastrointestinal toxicity of rofe-coxib and naproxen in patients with rheumatoid arthritis. *New England Journal of Medicine* **343** (21), 1520–1528.

Budd, K. (1994) Chronic pain – challenge and response. *Drugs* **47** (Suppl. 1), 33–38.

Burns-Cox, N., Campbell, W.B., Nimmen, B.A.J., Vercaeren, P.M.K. & Lucarotti, M. (1997) Surgical care and outcome for patients in their nineties. *British Journal of Surgery* **84** (4), 496–498.

Cleeland, C., Gonin, R., Hatfield, A.K., et al. (1994) Pain and its treat-ment in outpatients with metastatic cancer. *New England Journal of Medicine* **330**, 592–596.

Closs, J. (1994) Pain in elderly patients: a neglected phenomenon? *Journal of Advanced Nursing* **19** (6), 1072–1081.

Closs, J., Barr, B., Briggs, M., Cash, K. & Seers, K. (2004) A compari-son of five pain assessment scales for nursing home residents with varying degrees of cognitive impairment. *Journal of Pain and Symptom Management* **27** (3), 196–205.

Dalton, J.A. & McNaull, F. (1998) A call for standardizing the clinical rating of pain intensity using a 0 to 10 rating scale. *Cancer Nurse* **21**, 46–49.

Davis, M.A. (1988) Epidemiology of osteoarthritism. *Clinics of Geri-atric Medicine* **4**, 241–255.

Dean, M. (2004) Opioids in renal failure and dialysis patients. *Journal of Pain and Symptom Management* **28** (5), 497–504.

Decker, S.A. & Perry, A.G. (2003) The development and testing of the PATCOA to assess pain in confused older adults. *Pain Management Nursing* **4** (2), 77–86.

Desbiens, N.A. & Mueller-Rizner, N. (2000) How well do surrogates assess the pain of seriously ill patients? *Critical Care Medicine* **28** (5), 1347–1352.

Desbiens, N.A. & Wu, A.W. (2000) Pain and suffering in seriously ill hospitalized patients. *Journal of the American Geriatric Society* **48** (Suppl. 5), S183–S186.

Dessein, P.H., Shipton, E.A. & Budd, K. (1999) Oral low-dose gluco-corticosteroids as compared with intravenous methylprednisolone pulses in the treatment of rheumatoid arthritis. *Rheumatology* **38** (12), 1304–1305.

Dessein, P.H., Shipton, E.A. & Budd, K. (2000) Nociceptive and non-nociceptive rheumatological pain: recent developments in the understanding of pathophysiology and management in rheumatoid arthritis and fibromyalgia. *Pain Reviews* **7** (2), 67–79.

Dierking, G., Duedahl, T.H., Rasmussen, M.L., et al. (2004) Effects of gabapentin on postoperative morphine consumption and pain after abdominal hysterectomy: a randomized, double-blind trial. *Acta Anaesthesiologica Scandinavica* **48** (3), 322–327.

Downe-Wamboldt, B.L. & Melanson, P.M. (1998) A causal model of coping and well-being in elderly people with arthritis. *Journal of Advanced Nursing* **27** (6), 1109–1116.

Emery, P., Zeidler, H. & Kvien, T. (1999) Celecoxib vs diclofenac in long term management of rheumatoid arthritis. *The Lancet* **354**, 2106–2111.

FDA Advisory Committee (2001) *Cardiovascular Safety of Rofecoxib.* Food and Drug Administration, Rockville, Maryland.

Feldt, K.S. (2000) The checklist of nonverbal pain indicators (CNPI). *Pain Management Nursing* **1** (1), 13–21.

Ferrell, B.A. (1996) Overview of ageing and pain. In: Ferrell, B.R. & Ferrell, B.A. (eds) *Pain in the Elderly*. IASP Press, Seattle, pp. 1–10.

Ferrell, B.A., Ferrell, B.R. & Rivera, L. (1995) Pain in cognitively impaired nursing home patients. *Journal of Pain and Symptom Management* **10** (8), 591–598.

Ferrell, B.R. & Ferrell, B.A. (1996) An international perspective on pain in the elderly. In: Ferrell, B.R. & Ferrell, B.A. (eds) *Pain in the Elderly*. IASP Press, Seattle, pp. 119–130.

Foley, K. (1994) Pain in the elderly. In: Hazzard, W.R., Bierman, E.L., Blass, J.P., Ettinger, W.H. Jr. & Halter, J.B. (eds) *Principals of Geriatric Medicine and Gerontology*. McGraw-Hill, New York.

Fries, J. & Bruce, B. (2003) Rates of serious GI events from low dose use of acetylsalicylic acid, acetamophen and ibuprofen in patients with osteoarthritis and rheumatoid arthritis. *Journal of Rheumatology* **30** (10), 2226–2233.

Fuchs-Lacelle, S. & Hadjistavropoulos, T. (2004) Development and preliminary validation of the pain assessment checklist for seniors with limited ability to communicate (PACSLAC). *Pain Management Nursing* **5** (1), 37–49.

Gagliese, L. & Katz, J. (2003) Age differences in postoperative pain are scale dependent: a comparison of measures of pain intensity and quality in younger and older surgical patients. *Pain* **103** (1–2), 11–20.

Gagliese, L. & Melzack, R. (1997) Chronic pain in elderly people. *Pain* **70** (1) 3–14.

Gibson, S.J. & Helme, R.D. (2001) Age-related differences in pain perception and report. *Clinical Geriatric Medicine* **17**, 433–456.

Gillespie, L.D., Gillespie, W.J. & Robertson, M.C. (2002) *Interventions for Preventing Falls in Elderly People (Cochrane Review). The Cochrane Library, Issue 2.* Update Software, Oxford.

Goldstein, J.L., Kivitz, A.J., Verburg, K.M., Recker, D.P., Palmer, R.C. & Kent, J.C. (2003) A comparison of the upper gastrointestinal mucosal effects of valdecoxib, naproxen, naproxen and placebo in healthy elderly subjects. *Alimentary Pharmacology and Therapeutics* **18**, 125–132.

Griffin, M.R., Ray, W.A. & Schaffner, W. (1988) Non-steroidal antiinflammatory drug use and death from peptic ulcer in elderly patients. *Annals of Internal Medicine* **109**, 359–363.

Hanks-Bell, M., Halvey, K. & Paice, J.A. (2004) Pain assessment and management in ageing. *Online Journal of Issues in Nursing* **9** (3). Available at www.nursingworld.org/ojin/topic21/tpc21_6.htm, accessed September 2005.

Harstall, C. (2003) How prevalent is chronic pain? *Pain: Clinical Updates. International Association for the Study of Pain* **11** (2), 1–4.

Helme, R.D. (2001) Chronic pain management in older people. *European Journal of Pain* **5** (Suppl. A), 31–36.

Helme, R.D. & Gibson, S.J. (2001) The epidemiology of pain in elderly people. *Clinics in Geriatric Medicine* **17** (3), 417–431.

Helme, R.D., Andrews, P.V. & Allen, F. (1992) Medication use by elderly people resident in public housing in Melbourne. *Proceedings of the Australian Association of Gerontology* **27**, 30–33.

Henry, D., Dobson, A. & Turner, C. (1993) Variability and the risk of major gastrointestinal complications from non aspirin NSAIDs. *Gastroenterology* **105**, 1078–1088.

Hernandez-Diaz, S. & Rodriguez, L.A.G. (2000) Association between NSAIDs and upper GI tract bleeeding/perforation. *Archives of Internal Medicine* **160**, 2093–2099.

Herr, K. (2002) Pain assessment in cognitively impaired older adults. *American Journal of Nursing* **102** (12), 65–68.

Herr, K.A. & Mobily, P.R. (1993) Comparison of selected pain assessment tools for use with the elderly. *Applied Nursing Research* **6**, 39–46.

Hippisley Cox, J. & Coupland, C. (2005) Risk of myocardial infarction in patients taking cyclo-oxygenase-2 inhibitors or conventional non-steroidal anti-inflammatory drugs: population based nested case-control analysis. *British Medical Journal* **330** (11), 1366.

Hirshberg, B., Mordechi, M., Schlesinger, O. & Rubinow, A. (2000) Safety of low dose methotrexate in elderly patients with rheumatoid arthritis. *Postgraduate Medical Journal* **76** (Dec), 787–798.

Hurley, A.C., Volicer, B.J., Hanrahan, S.H. & Volicer, L. (1992) Assessment of discomfort in advanced Alzheimer patients. *Research in Nursing and Health* **15** (3), 69–377.

Hylek, E.M., Heiman, H., Skates, S.J., Sheehan, M.A. & Singer, D.E. (1998) Acetaminophen and other risk factors for excessive warfarin anticoagulation. *JAMA* **279**, 657–662.

Jakobsson, U. & Hallberg, I.R. (2002) Pain and quality of life among older people with rheumatoid arthritis and/or osteoarthritis: a literature review. *Journal of Clinical Nursing* **11**, 430–443.

Jensen, M.P., Karoly, P. & Braver, S. (1986) The measurement of clinical pain intensity: a comparison of six methods. *Pain* **27**, 117–126.

Kassalainen, S. & Crook, J. (2004) An exploration of seniors' ability to report pain. *Clinical Nursing Research* **13** (3), 199–215.

Kavanaugh, A.F. (1997) Rheumatoid arthritis in the elderly: is it a different disease? The *American Journal of Medicine* **103** (6), 40S–48S.

Kennedy, D. & Small, R. (1997) Analgesics and elderly patients. *Pain Clinic Perspectives* **7** (6), 14–15.

Kidd, B.L. (2002) Nociceptive mechanisms in the inflammatory arthropathies. Pain. In: Giamberadino, M.A. (ed.) *An Updated Review: Refresher Course Syllabus*. IASP Press, Seattle.

Kitte, F.J. (1966) The effects of limitation of activity upon the human body. *JAMA* **196**, 117–122.

Konttinen, R.A., Kemppinen, Y.T., Segerberg, P., et al. (1994) Peripheral and spinal neural mechanisms in arthritis, with particular reference to treatment of inflammation and pain. *Arthritis and Rheumatism* **37** (7),965–982.

Kovach, C.R., Noonan, P.E., Griffie, J., Muchka, S. & Weissman, D.E. (2002) The assessment of discomfort in dementia protocol. *Pain Management Nursing* **3** (1), 16–27.

Lambert, V.A., Lambert, C.E., Kipple, G.L. & Mewshaw, E.A. (1990) Relationship among hardiness, social supports, severity of illness and psychological well being in women with rheumatoid arthritis. *Health Care for Women International* **11**, 159–173.

Langman, M., Weil, J., Wainwright, P., et al. (1994) Risks of bleeding peptic ulcer with individual NSAIDs. *The Lancet* **343** (May), 1075–1078.

Lee, D. & Weinblatt, M. (2001) Rheumatoid arthritis. *The Lancet* **358**, 903–911.

Leese, P.T., Recker, D.P. & Kent, J.D. (2003) The COX-2 selective inhibitor, valdecoxib, does not impair platelet function in the elderly: results of a randomized controlled trial. *Journal of Clinical Pharmacology* **43** (5), 504–513.

Lefebvre-Chapiro, S., Trivalle, C., Legrain, S., Feteanu, D. & Sebag-Lanoe, R. (2001) The DOLOPLUS 2 scale – evaluating pain in the elderly. *European Journal of Palliative Care* **8** (5), 191–194. See www.doloplus.com, accessed October 2005.

Manfredi, P.L., Breuer, B., Meier, D.E. & Libow, L. (2003) Pain assessment in elderly patients with severe dementia. *Journal of Pain and Symptom Management* **25** (1), 48–52.

Martin, B. & Ali, B. (2002) Regional nerve block in fractured neck of femur. *Emergency Medicine Journal* **19**, 144–145.

McCaffery, M. & Beebe, A. (1994) *Pain: Clinical Manual for Nursing Practice*. Mosby, London.

McCaffery, R. & Freeman, E. (2003) Effect of music on chronic osteoarthritis pain in older people. *Journal of Advanced Nursing* **44** (5), 517–524.

McQuay, H., Carrol, D., Jadad, A.R., Wiffen, P. & Moore, A. (1995) Anticonvulsant drugs for management of pain: a systematic review. *British Medical Journal* **311**, 1047–1052.

Merck (2005) *The Merck Manual of Geriatrics*. Section 7 Musculoskeletal Disorders, Chapter 52 Rheumatic Diseases, Rheumatoid Arthritis. Available at www.merck.com/mrkshared/mmg/sec7/ch52/ch52a.jsp, accessed October 2005.

Moore, R.A. & Phillips, C.J. (1999) Cost of NSAID adverse effects to the UK National Health Service. *Journal of Medical Economics* **2**, 45–55.

Morrison, R.S. & Siu, A.L. (2000) A comparison of pain and its treatment in advanced dementia and cognitively intact patients with hip fracture. *Journal of Pain and Symptom Management* **19** (4), 240–248.

National Guideline Clearinghouse (2004) *Clinical Practice Guideline for the Management of Rheumatoid Arthritis*. Available at www.guideline.gov, accessed October 2005.

National Institute for Health and Clinical Excellence (2001) *Osteoarthritis and Rheumatoid Arthritis – Cox II Inhibitors (No. 27)*. See www.nice.org.uk/page.aspx?o, accessed October 2005.

Nicholas, J. (1994) Physical modalities in rheumatological rehabilitation. *Archives of Physical Medicine and Rehabilitation* **75** (9), 994–1001.

Office for National Statistics (2002) Population estimates for data on age structure and gender. Available at www.statistics.gov.uk, accessed September 2005.

Prodigy (2005) *Prodigy Guidance – Rheumatoid Arthritis*. Available at www.prodigy.nhs.uk/indexmain.asp, accessed October 2005.

Reuben, S.S., Steinberg, R.B., Maciolek, H. & Joshi, W. (2002) Preoperative administration of controlled-release oxycodone for the management of pain after ambulatory laparoscopic tubal ligation surgery. *Journal of Clinical Anesthesia* **14** (3), 223–227.

Robinson, S. & Benson, G. (2002) Warmed blankets: an intervention to promote comfort for elderly hospitalized patients. *Geriatric Nursing* **23** (6), 320–323.

Rosenthal, N.R., Silverfield, J.C., Wu, S.-C., Jordan, D. & Kamin, M. (2004) Tramadol/acetaminophen combination tablets for the treatment of pain associated with osteoarthritis flare in an elderly patient population. *Journal of the American Geriatrics Society* **52** (3), 374–380.

Sack, K. (1995) Osteoarthritis – a continuing challenge. *Western Journal of Medicine* **163**, 579–586.

Savage, R. (2005) Cyclo-oxygenase-2 inhibitors: when should they be used in the elderly. *Drugs and Aging* **22** (3), 185–200.

Schwameder, H., Roithner, R., Muller, E., Niessen, W. & Raschner, C. (1999) Knee joint forces during downhill walking with hiking poles. *Journal of Sports Sciences* **17** (12), 969–978.

Schofield, P. (2005) *Beyond Pain*. John Wiley, London.

Schofield, P., Dunham, M. & Black, C. (2005) *Older People – Managing Their Pain in the Community Setting*. Available at www.jcn.co.uk/journal.asp?monthnum=09&yearnum=2005&type=search&articleid=844.

Shipton, E.A. (1999) Secondary analgesics (Part 1). In: Shipton, E.A. (ed.) *Pain – Acute and Chronic*. Arnold, London, pp. 93–107.

Silverstein, F.E., Faich, G., Goldstein, J.L., et al. (2000) Gastrointestinal toxicity with celecoxib vs NSAIDs for osteoarthritis and rheumatoid arthritis. *JAMA* **284** (10), 1247–1255.

Simons, W. & Malabar, R. (1995) Assessing pain in elderly patients who cannot respond verbally. *Journal of Advanced Nursing* **22** (4), 663–669.

Snow, A.L., Weber, J.B., O'Malley, K.J., et al. (2004) NOPPAIN: a nursing assistant-administered pain assessment instrument for use in dementia. *Dementia Geriatric Cognitive Disorders* **17** (3), 240–246.

Stenstrom, C.H. (1994) Home exercise in rheumatoid arthritis functional class II: goal setting versus pain attention. *Journal of Rheumatology* **21**, 627–631.

Strong, J., Unruh, A.M., Wright, A. & Baxter, G.D. (2002) *Pain: Textbook for Therapists*. Churchill Livingstone, Edinburgh.

SUPPORT Investigators (1995) A controlled trial to improve outcomes for seriously ill hospitalized patients: study to understand prognoses and preferences for outcomes and risks of treatments (SUPPORT). *JAMA* **274**, 20.

Taha, J.M. & Tew, J.M. Jr. (1996) Comparison of surgical treatments for trigeminal neuralgia: reevaluation of radiofrequency rhizotomy. *Neurosurgery* **38**, 865–871.

Thomas, E., Peat, G., Harris, L., Wilkie, R. & Croft, P.R. (2004) The prevalence of pain and pain interference in a general population of older adults. *Pain* **110**, 361–368.

Villanueva, M.R., Smith, T.L., Erickson, J.S., Lee, A.C. & Singer, C.M. (2003) Pain assessment for the dementing elderly (PADE): reliability and validity of a new measure. *Journal of the American Medical Directors Association* **4** (1), 1–8.

Visser, E., Graatsma, H. & Stricker, B. (2002) Contraindicated NSAIDs are frequently prescribed to elderly patients with peptic ulcer disease. *British Journal of Clinical Pharmacology* **53** (2), 183–188.

Walker, J.S. (2001) Anti-inflammatory effects of κ-opioids: relevance to rheumatoid arthritis. *Pain Reviews* **8** (3–4), 113–119.

Warden, V., Hurley, A.C. & Volicer, L. (2003) Development and psychometric evaluation of the pain assessment in advanced dementia (PAINAD) scale. *Journal of the American Medical Directors Association* **4** (1), 9–15.

Weiner, D.K., Herr, K. & Rudy, T. (2002) *Persistent Pain in Older Adults. An Interdisciplinary Guide for Treatment.* Springer, New York. See www.americangeriatrics.org/products/positionpapers/JGS5071. pdf, accessed October 2005.

World Health Organization (2004) Ageing pain and cancer: the role of geriatrics, oncology and palliative care. *Cancer Pain Release* 17 (1&2). See www.whocancerpain.wisc.edu/eng/17_1-2/ interview.html, accessed October 2005.

The Organisation of Pain Management Services

INTRODUCTION

This chapter is different from previous chapters in that it focuses primarily on pain services and organisations that contribute to the management of pain. It has a similar structure in that it starts by considering the management of acute pain, but rather than the individual, it will focus on the services and people that might be involved in the provision of a hospital acute pain team (APT). The following section considers services available for the management of chronic pain both in hospital and in the community, such as chronic pain clinics. There follows a section on the provision of palliative care services. Patient, professional and organisational barriers are explored before considering some of the global issues and in particular policies that influence the availability of adequate pain relief. It is not by accident that the penultimate section of this book reflects on the ethical and legal parameters that influence our practice.

Nurses have a pivotal role to play in the organisation and delivery of pain management. The British Pain Society has published an excellent document, which identifies a progressive range of competencies, from novice to expert, for nurses working in pain management (British Pain Society 2002). It also includes chapters on different pain services and the nursing contribution.

LEARNING OBJECTIVES

❏ Identify which services might be available for patients experiencing acute and chronic pain
❏ Describe the role of different health care professionals and their contribution to the management of pain
❏ Recognise the ethical and legal issues that might arise when managing pain

---

> **Box 8.1 Acute pain teams (APTs) in English hospitals**
>
> A survey was carried out in 2002 by McDonnell et al. (2003) to ascertain the provision of multidisciplinary acute pain teams (APTs) in English hospitals performing adult in-patient surgery. A response rate of 86% ($n = 226$) was achieved after written and telephone reminders. The survey indicated that 84% of respondents had an APT in their hospital. However, some hospitals still had no team and recent evidence indicates that some APTs face financial difficulties and have a 'token' service only.

ACUTE PAIN TEAMS (APTs)

Acute pain is extremely common in hospitals and most often occurs after surgery. Other conditions such as acute low back pain, trauma, burns and many medical conditions (e.g. myocardial infarction, acute pancreatitis and sickle cell disease) also give rise to acute pain. In the early 1990s the Royal College of Surgeons of England and the College of Anaesthetists produced recommendations for the provision of multidisciplinary teams in hospitals to provide acute pain services (Royal College of Surgeons of England and College of Anaesthetists 1990). The majority of hospitals in England now provide this service (see Box 8.1). Specialist nurses have an important role within these teams and usually work alongside staff from other disciplines, such as anaesthetists, psychologists, physiotherapists and pharmacists.

APTs have been associated with introduction of the more advanced technical approaches such as patient controlled analgesia (PCA) and epidurals. Some hospitals may organise these interventions through their APT, whilst others include them as a routine part of care without referral to the APT. Epidural analgesics require appropriate resources (pumps, prepared pharmacological packs, trained staff and observation) and hospital variation results in some patients receiving epidural analgesia only in high dependency areas, or intensive care, whilst other hospitals might care for such patients on the ward.

The use of other interventions such as Entonox and transcutaneous electrical nerve stimulation (TENS) is often incorporated into the patient's care if appropriate. A typical day for a clinical nurse specialist working for an APT might include the following:

- A visit to a patient with an epidural that does not seem to be working
- A young child has been admitted following a fall from a swing and seems very distressed; he needs a PCA to be set up
- A young man who was admitted in the night with fractured ribs has intense pain – an assessment is needed to plan his care and possibly arrange an anaesthetist to put in an epidural for a couple of days
- Team meeting with anaesthetist and pharmacist to discuss the possibility of removing a 'co-drug' from the prescribing formulary because it is not particularly effective as an analgesic
- Teaching a seminar on 'acute pain' with a group of junior doctors
- Teaching session and assessment with two new staff nurses not familiar with the hospital PCA machine
- Organising a pain audit with the Accident and Emergency department

One of the key activities of an APT is the provision of education for hospital staff. The importance of accurate assessment and documentation as well as teaching staff how to manage acute pain, using newer technologies, is often a core part of the APT's activity. Specific assessment charts might be used which also provide advice on increasing or decreasing the analgesia available to patients, depending on their pain score (at rest and on movement) and vital signs.

In the same way that we assess pain in order to gain an understanding of how well we are doing with our interventions, a service also needs to be assessed in order to measure the quality of the service. This is usually through 'clinical audit' and is an essential activity of an APT. Measurable standards are set and the audit measures whether these standards have been achieved. Below are examples of standards and the parallel audit activity:

Standard
- No patient will have an acute pain score of >6 on a 0–10 scale on two successive assessments.
- Every postoperative patient will have a pain assessment chart with a pain score documented within the past 4 hours.

Audit
- Count how many patients score >6 during the time of their hospital admission.
- How many patients have a pain assessment chart *and* a pain score has been documented in the past 4 hours?

Clinical audit is not a one-off activity but forms part of a cycle (McCleod 2002):

- Identify the clinical problem
- Develop standards as a benchmark
- Conduct the audit
- Compare results with the standard
- Implement a change (e.g. education)
- Evaluate the impact of change

Coleman & Booker-Milburn (1996) undertook an audit to assess the influence of the acute pain nurse who conducted regular pain rounds and teaching of staff. The provision of such nursing led to a reduction in the side effects of epidural analgesia and improvement in pain relief with PCA.

Sometimes there is confusion over what constitutes 'research' and what is 'audit'. It is helpful to think that 'research is finding out what you should be doing; audit is whether you are doing what you ought to be doing' (Wilson et al. 1999).

PALLIATIVE CARE SERVICES

Palliative care has been shown to be effective at improving symptom control and quality of life in patients with cancer as well as long-term conditions (DoH 2005).

> 'Palliative care seeks to prevent, relieve, reduce, or soothe the symptoms of disease or disorder without effecting a cure. Palliative care in this broad sense is not restricted to those dying or those enrolled in a hospice program. It attends closely to the emotional, spiritual, and practical needs and goals of patients and those close to them.' (Field & Cassel 1997)

Cancer continues to afflict millions of people, and whilst for many this disease curtails their longevity, many gain remission and lead full and active lives. The fear of pain in advanced cancer is one of the most cited anxieties reported by sufferers and yet there is no need to suffer needless pain (Fine 1999). Whilst many patients experiencing cancer do not require specialist pain services, between 10 and 15% do. This may be provided in their own homes by specialist nurses, such as those of the Marie Curie charity, or they may require admission to a hospice. Many hospitals have their own palliative care team which provides specialist services for patients with cancer. A team might consist of:

- A consultant in palliation
- Specialist nurse
- Clinical psychologist
- Specialist registrar or anaesthetists with specialist expertise, e.g. neural blocks
- Chaplain

Liaison between the APT, palliative care team and the patient's GP is essential to ensure patients are referred to such services in a timely manner (see Box 8.2). The case study of Joanne demonstrates the complexity of such care and highlights the need for good communication between the different professionals at this time. The fear and anxiety likely to accompany these events can heighten the experience of pain.

Case study

Joanne, aged 38, was recently admitted for a resection of her colon following the discovery of a cancerous growth in her large bowel. She is a young woman with two pre-school children as well as a part-time job at the local supermarket. The shock of major surgery and the diagnosis of cancer had catapulted her life into turmoil. A computer-assisted tomography (CAT) scan revealed extensive metastatic spread of the disease to her spine and other organs. Joanne had noticed a constant low backache for the past few months but put it down to tiredness and always bending down. The APT had suggested that a referral be made to the palliative care service.

> **Box 8.2 Management of pain in palliative care**
>
> In a study by Bostrom et al. (2004), 30 Swedish patients with cancer were interviewed in order to gain an understanding of how patients with cancer-related pain in palliative care perceived the management of their pain. Three main categories emerged: communication, planning and trust. The opportunity for patients to discuss their pain and its management appeared to have occurred late in the disease process, mostly not until coming into contact with a palliative care team. This study highlights the importance of early referral to specialist services and the need for continual assessment and communication between patients and those providing services.

To ensure that Joanne receives optimal care the following steps should be taken:

- Referral by the surgical team to the palliative care service for specialist advice
- All communication should be copied to Joanne's GP to ensure he/she is aware
- The inclusion of family or close friends

The hospice

The 'hospice movement' was built upon the pioneering work of Dame Ciceley Saunders who trained as a nurse and a doctor and worked at St. Joseph's Hospice in the East End of London. The observation of 900 dying patients at St. Joseph's Hospice gave her data to argue that opioids were not addictive, that tolerance was not a problem and that giving morphine orally worked by relieving pain, not by merely masking it (Seymour et al. 2005). The focus of hospice care is on maintaining quality of life, including relief from pain and other distressing symptoms, while integrating medical, psychological and spiritual aspects of care. The emphasis is on living an active life and support for families during the patient's illness and in bereavement. The delivery of care can be in the patient's home or a dedicated unit. Palliative and hospice care are often underpinned by the same philosophy and approach. Higginson et al. (2003) conducted a study to determine the effects of palliative care and hospice care teams (PCHCT) on end-of-life experiences. In 44 studies they identified five different types of teams:

(1) Home care (22)
(2) Hospital-based (9)
(3) Combined home/hospital care (4)
(4) Inpatient units (3)
(5) Integrated teams (6)

They remarked on the wide variation in the teams, but their data analysis suggested that evidence of benefit was strongest for home care.

One of the most important activities of palliative and hospice care teams is that they often coordinate care and improve communication between professionals and the individual patient and family. Many of the barriers mentioned in previous chapters are relevant, but one of the most important considerations identified by patients experiencing cancer pain is communication between the patient and professionals (Ashby & Dowding 2001; Bostrom et al. 2004).

CHRONIC PAIN SERVICES

In the UK, and indeed worldwide, specialist services have evolved to help people suffering with chronic pain. There are two main services: the chronic pain clinic and chronic pain programmes. People experiencing chronic pain have been found to visit their GP up to five times more often than other patients, resulting in nearly 5 million appointments every year, but only a few get referred to specialist services. The British Pain Society has published guidelines on setting up chronic pain services in primary care (see Box 8.3).

Box 8.3 *A Practical Guide to the Provision of Chronic Pain Services for Adults in Primary Care* (British Pain Society and Royal College of General Practitioners 2004)

This practical document aims to help health care professionals, and in particular nurses, set up chronic pain services in primary care. Key topics are:

- Assessing pain management in primary care practices
- Patient assessment
- Aims and liaison in primary care
- When to refer
- Educational pain management courses in the UK
- Example leaflets for patients

Chronic pain clinic

Pain clinics have evolved to provide a full assessment of a patient with a persisting pain problem, particularly when no curative treatment is available. In general terms these are 'specialist chronic pain services', often hospital based and led by a consultant. Referral is usually made from a GP, consultant within a hospital or trust or the APT. Many patients attending pain clinics, especially those referred by other specialists, will already have an established medical diagnosis. In the UK there have been concerns about long waiting lists (18 months or longer) and poor local provision, requiring patients to travel excessive distances. Disappointingly these inadequacies were pointed out several years ago and the situation shows little improvement (see Box 8.4). Interventions range from nerve blocks and epidurals to lifestyle education. Nicholas (2004) undertakes a comprehensive review of factors associated with referral to chronic pain clinics, interventions and anticipated outcomes.

Pain management programmes

These are variations of the above but usually have a programme that requires the patient to attend either on an outpatient or on an in-patient basis. They are usually one week to one month in duration and very intensive. The intensive programmes appear to have more benefits than non-intensive ones. They are multidisciplinary and many include a medical consultant, physiotherapist, occupational therapist, nurse, pharmacist and clinical psychologist. The emphasis is on helping patients live and cope with their pain rather than a cure. Encouraging the cessation or reduction of medication is important and training in self-help and coping skills, including cognitive behavioural therapy, usually takes a prominent role.

BARRIERS TO EFFECTIVE PAIN MANAGEMENT – PATIENT, PROFESSIONAL AND ORGANISATIONAL

Patient barriers

Patients may not achieve adequate analgesia because they are extremely reluctant to take strong medication, even when a regime that includes a strong opioid has proved to be effective and the side effects manageable. The following are often highlighted as examples of patient concerns that need to be addressed:

- Patients may expect pain and have poor expectations of treatment.
- Patients often do not realise that pain can contribute to harmful side effects, especially if palliative surgery has been necessary.
- They may have heard stories that overemphasise harmful drug side effects. Patients are often reluctant to trouble the 'busy nurses'.
- If they have cancer they may worry that these stronger drugs may not work at the end if they start taking them now.
- They may fear being seen as not coping or being a nuisance.
- Patients may think their pain needs to be severe to warrant treatment.
- Opioids, particularly morphine, have a poor image and can be seen as 'death' drugs.
- Even patients with end stage cancer may fear addiction or fear being labeled as an 'addict'.
- Side effects may have been allowed to become intolerable before treatment to overcome these was started and then patients may perceive the side effects as being worse than the pain.
- They may also perceive strong opioids to be ineffective if they have not been titrated to effect or when one proves unsuitable for an individual patient and an alternative opioid is never tried.

Professional barriers

When trying to ensure the effective management of pain with people who have cancer it is salient to be aware of some of the professional and organisational barriers that might impede a timely referral to palliative care services (Box 8.5). Sometimes professionals are reluctant to relinquish the care of their patient to

---

Box 8.5 Barriers to pain management

A total of 1015 registered nurses completed a 21-item survey examining barriers to pain management. More than one third of the respondents indicated they had encountered at least one barrier to providing optimal relief, including insufficient co-operation by physicians and inadequate prescription of analgesic medications. (See Van Niekerk & Martin 2003.)

---

another service as they may feel they are able to manage the patient's symptoms. In the previous case study it might be unwillingness, on behalf of the surgical team, to facilitate the referral, whereas in the community a GP may be reluctant to refer to specialists, fearing it might fragment care and possibly overwhelm the family. In each case the needs of the patient and his or her family must be the prime consideration and good communication, between all parties, is paramount. If there are concerns that the patient continues to experience unrelieved pain, then this should be documented. Informal contact with the service may help smooth the way.

Waiting for a referral can be frustrating, as sometimes the original prescription for analgesics is no longer sufficient and the patient experiences pain. Nurses often find themselves in the invidious position of finding a patient who is in pain due to an inadequate prescription and feeling that they cannot do anything about it. The following might be helpful in negotiating a change of prescription:

- Ensure the optimum prescribed analgesic(s) have been given.
- Regular assessment and documentation of pain should illustrate the inadequacy.
- When presenting a request for an increase/change in prescription, give the vital signs as well as the current pain score.
- Suggest the change – perhaps adding in an oral opioid for breakthrough pain or a regular NSAID.
- Suggest the change for a trial period, with a time set for review.

There are a number of other barriers that have been well reported over the years:

- Lack of knowledge and appropriate attitudes
- Lack of assessment and documentation

Box 8.6 *Observation of Pain Assessment and Management – The Complexities of Clinical Practice* (Manias et al. 2002)

An observational study of 12 registered nurses in Australia managing patient pain found some important barriers that impeded good care:

- **Interruptions** – antibiotics, telephone, relatives, student nurses
- **Attending cues** – tended to be vigilant when doing observations but at other times when patients expressed pain they would acknowledge the statement but not follow up
- **Interpretation** – tended to focus on incisional pain and ignore other sources of pain discomfort. Continued to try to take blood despite obvious distress
- **Competing demands** – doctors requiring patient to be in uncomfortable position; junior doctors insisted on dressing protocol but it was uncomfortable – nurse went to registrar

---

- Concerns about addiction and respiratory depression
- Lack of time

As well as professional barriers the clinical environment produces organisational barriers (see Box 8.6). The next section considers how the organisation might impede effective pain management.

Organisational barriers

The lack of accountability in an organisation has figured as one of the main reasons pain was inadequately managed, as long ago as 1977 (Fagerhaugh & Strauss 1977). Quite often no one individual seems to take responsibility, which often means the patient continues to experience pain. Nurses can be the key to ensuring this is prevented by taking such responsibility.

Hospital policies may inadvertently hinder the timely delivery of opioids: for instance, hospital policy insisting on two trained nurses to check controlled drugs when this is not a legal requirement. The policy can appear nonsensical when you consider that more hazardous drugs such as digoxin, for which there is no reversal agent, are routinely single checked. Also the practice of insisting that a medication such as oral morphine syrup (10 mg in 5 ml, which is not a controlled drug) only be stored in the controlled drug cupboard rather than along with other easily available analgesia on the ward drug trolley.

Other factors such as inadequate resources and funding may limit specialist pain services or the number of PCAs available. Tackling this can be difficult, but often audit data can highlight the problems and act as a catalyst for resources. The following sections describe some of the national and international organisations that are endeavouring to improve the management of pain.

PROFESSIONAL ORGANISATIONS

There are a number of organisations that champion for improved pain management not only for individuals in their own countries but also for people whose countries may have no services for pain management or even analgesics. There are many different organisations interested in promoting the improvement of pain and we have chosen three to illustrate their work and initiatives. This is to give you a wider perspective and to see how you as an individual can link to the larger picture.

British organisations

The Royal College of Nursing has a pain special interest group known as the Pain Forum (Pain Points) which runs a number of study days and produces a regular newsletter. Further information can be obtained from the RCN website www.rcn.org.uk/members/resources (accessed October 2005).

The Pain Network is a UK organisation developed by nurses to promote awareness and provide support for members regarding pain management. It is a network that is organised into ten regions, each with its own educational support group. A newsletter is produced four times a year. Further information can be found on their website www.painnetwork.co.uk/info.asp (accessed October 2005).

The British Pain Society states that it is 'an alliance of professionals advancing the understanding and management of pain for the benefit of patients'. It began in 1979 as the Intractable Pain Society of Great Britain and Ireland with a membership limited primarily to anaesthetists managing pain clinics. Over time, the membership of the Society became more and more multidisciplinary, and in 1988 the Society changed its name to the Pain Society and the British Pain Society in 2004. Membership continues to grow and the Society's work covers a range of activities, from close work with patient groups lobbying parliament for better pain services to the production of recommendations for professionals regarding pain management. See www. britishpainsociety.org (accessed October 2005).

International associations

The International Association for the Study of Pain (IASP) is the largest multidisciplinary international association in the field of pain. Founded in 1973, IASP is a non-profit professional organisation dedicated to furthering research on pain and improving the care of patients with pain. Membership of IASP is open to scientists, physicians, dentists, psychologists, nurses, physical therapists and other health professionals actively engaged in pain research and to those who have special interest in the diagnosis and treatment of pain. Currently IASP has more than 6,500 individual members from over 100 countries. In the UK the British Pain Society is a member chapter. IASP has an excellent website (www.iasp-pain.org/index.html, accessed October 2005) and holds a triennial congress attracting over 6,000 delegates.

Europe also has a multidisciplinary professional organisation in the field of pain science and medicine, made up of the 28 European chapters of IASP. Established in 1993, the European Federation of IASP Chapters (EFIC) has 28 constituent chapters representing close to 15,000 scientists, physicians, nurses, physiotherapists, psychologists and other health care professionals across Europe who study pain and treat patients in pain. EFIC's aims are to advance research, education, clinical management and professional practice related to pain, and to serve as an authoritative, scientifically based resource concerning policy issues related to pain and its management. They too are very active in bringing the inadequacies of pain management to the attention of the public, professionals, government and the wider world. Each year a 'Week Against Pain' is organised and details can be found on the website www.efic.org (accessed October 2005).

The World Health Organization (WHO) has been proactive in lobbying for better pain relief on a number of fronts over many years. Some of these endeavours include:

- The WHO three-step analgesia ladder (WHO 1996)
- Support of 'Global Day Against Pain' (11 October 2004, Geneva; see below)
- Palliative care and symptom management guidelines for people living with HIV/AIDS (WHO 2004)
- *Cancer Pain Release* is part of the WHO's global communications programme to improve cancer pain control and palliative and supportive care (see www.whocancerpain.wisc.edu, accessed October 2005)

In an effort to raise awareness of the inhumanity of pain and needless suffering, WHO collaborated with the British Pain Society in 2004 and held a 'Global Day Against Pain', running live satellite interviews with key leaders in the field of pain management and research, which was broadcast on the Internet. The organisation of this venture should not be underestimated and demonstrates the immense commitment the WHO has to removing some of the international barriers. Its motto for 2004 was 'the relief of pain should be a human right'.

GLOBAL PAIN POLICIES
During the course of this book we have guided you to consider the best evidence available to use when caring for an individual with pain. Within your own practice, be it on a ward, outpatient or even in a community setting, there will often be barriers to the effective delivery of care for people in pain. For instance, your hospital may require two nurses to check a controlled drug. This takes time and can increase the delay for patients waiting in pain for their analgesics. We would identify this as an 'organisational barrier' and encourage the collection of data to record the average time patients wait for analgesics, and then use these data to lobby for a change of policy, such as single nurse checking. Beyond our hospitals and communities there exist further barriers and these are often hidden in the international and global communities.

Pain and Policy Studies Group, University of Wisconsin
Barriers are often present as a result of national policies and it is in this area that the Pain and Policy Studies Group of the University of Wisconsin directs a considerable amount of its

activity (Gilson et al. 2005). It has produced some excellent statistics highlighting the inadequate consumption of opioids in different countries around the world. Some countries have such stringent policies regarding the import of opioids or narcotics that the medical need for people legitimately experiencing cancer or surgical pain is neglected. The national 'quota' for importing opioids is linked to each country's drug policy and clearly some governments might prefer not to import these drugs as they cannot be sure they will remain in safe hands.

The work of WHO would naturally fall into this global arena. As outlined earlier it has worked tirelessly to bring expertise from around the world to address issues of pain in cancer, often its focus being on helping people for whom health service infrastructures are poorly developed.

LEGAL AND ETHICAL CONSIDERATIONS

The care of people experiencing pain is often inextricably bound with ethical considerations. Health care professionals have a duty to relieve pain and so strong is this responsibility it is central to many of the mission statements espoused by their professional organisations (e.g. the Nursing and Midwifery Council (NMC), American Nursing Association, General Medical Council and the World Health Organization). The following section describes some of the ethical considerations that are particularly important when managing pain. See also Ferrell (2005) whose article provides ethical perspectives on pain and its management.

Responsibility and accountability

Central to the Nursing and Midwifery Council's *Code of Professional Conduct* (NMC 2004) is the concept of responsibility and accountability. Nearly 30 years ago Fagerhaugh & Strauss (1977) published the findings from their study of pain management. They made the salutary conclusion that the inadequacies they observed were primarily due to a lack of accountability. In acute pain management we often see accountability move from the surgeon, to the acute pain team, to the GP when the patient is discharged home. The nurse is in an ideal position to ensure that accountability remains transparent and that regular assessment and documentation takes place and is communicated to others.

Autonomy

This concerns autonomous decision-making in relation to your professional training and will rely upon your knowledge about pain management. A recent survey of 101 doctors and nurses in the UK found that they rated their undergraduate programme as the least helpful source of pain education (Coulling 2005). The inadequacies of pain education in the undergraduate curriculum have been reported in a variety of health professions across different countries, including nursing, pharmacy, occupational therapy and physical therapy. Whilst nurses should have an ethical responsibility to self-assess their own knowledge it is recognised that the profession also has a responsibility to ensure that appropriate education is included at pre-registration. Teaching pain management to undergraduates from a variety of health care professions is the way forward (Watt-Watson et al. 2004).

Beneficence

The principle of beneficence would suggest the responsibility of nurses to do good by helping people experiencing pain. Threats to beneficence might include undermedication, misconceptions about the nature of pain and failure of undergraduate curricula to adequately prepare the professionals who will be providing pain relief.

Non-maleficence

In its simplest form this is the notion of not inflicting harm on others and is sometimes referred to as 'double effect'. Through our endeavours to provide effective pain relief the effects of our interventions may precipitate unwanted side effects, such as nausea or constipation. Interestingly these are very troublesome to patients and yet health care professionals do not appear to have the same anxieties. On the contrary health care professionals always seem far more concerned with a mild level of sedation, for which the patient may well be grateful postoperatively! Nurses may have misplaced their concerns on the possibility of addiction or respiratory depression, which are very rare occurrences.

Box 8.7 Barriers to managing pain in the nursing home

In a statewide survey of all licensed Connecticut nursing homes in the USA (Tarzian & Hoffman 2005), 113 directors of nursing responded to a survey identifying barriers to providing pain management. The three most important barriers were identified as:

- Lack of knowledge among nursing home nurses
- Lack of knowledge among nursing home physicians
- Facility physicians' attitudes toward treating pain (including concerns about addiction or overdose)

Justice

Justice is concerned with equal treatment and the distribution of resources. The ability to care with equality and impartiality for an individual in pain is not supported by the research findings. Numerous papers highlight the differences in pain management according to patient characteristics such as sex, age and social class. A telephone survey of access to treatment for chronic pain found that access was influenced by ethnic background (Nguyen et al. 2005). Similarly older people may not receive good quality pain management when they are in a nursing home (see Box 8.7). This area continues to be a major challenge to the delivery of pain management.

Veracity

The rules of veracity are concerned with telling the truth, confidentiality and privacy. How truthful are we when we give an injection or remove a dressing that has adhered to the skin and say 'It won't hurt much'? Meanwhile the patient tightly squeezes his or her eyes closed, grimaces and holds his/her breath until we have finished. Telling the truth is central to gaining trust and forms one of the dominant threads in the nurse–patient relationship. Doctors may assume the responsibility for informing patients of the painful side effects of chemotherapy or a surgical procedure but it will be the nurse who sits alongside that patient in pain.

SUMMARY

The essential clinical skills required to promote effective pain management have been illustrated throughout the book. The management of pain does not rely solely on the nurse or the doctor, but often involves a range of people who work within a given context. Moving beyond our local environment we see a number of organisations active in the promotion of the effective management of pain. They might be lobbying members of parliament or providing additional studies where nurses and other health care professionals can learn more about pain. Beyond these organisations there is an international arena where pain continues to be discussed and solutions sought for enduring problems. The language may be different, but often the problems are the same. So we arrive in a global place and we think about how our individual countries help us to help others to manage pain. It is there that, perhaps, the greatest improvements can be made. When we come together to share our challenges, knowledge and skills we are usually better placed to understand and move forward. We hope this book will have provided you with the knowledge, skills and confidence to experience the same feeling.

REFERENCES

Ashby, M.E. & Dowding, C. (2001) Hospice care and patients' pain: communication between patients, relatives, nurses and doctors. *International Journal of Palliative Nursing* **7**, 58–67.

Bostrom, B., Sandh, M. & Lundberg, D. (2004) Cancer-related pain in palliative care: patients' perceptions of pain management. *Journal of Advanced Nursing* **45** (4), 410–419.

British Pain Society (2002) *Recommendations for Nurses Working in Pain Management*. Nursing Focus in Pain Management Working Party of the Pain Society. British Pain Society, London. Available at www.britishpainsociety.org/pub_pub.html, accessed October 2005.

British Pain Society and Royal College of General Practitioners (2004) *A Practical Guide to the Provision of Chronic Pain Services for Adults in Primary Care*. Available at www.britishpainsociety.org/pdf/napp_resourcepack.pdf, accessed October 2005.

Coleman, S.A. & Booker-Milburn, J. (1996) Audit of post-operative pain control: influence of a dedicated acute pain nurse. *Anaesthesia* **51** (12), 1093–1096.

Coulling, S. (2005) Nurses' and doctors' knowledge of pain after surgery. *Nursing Standard* **19** (34), 41–49.

Department of Health (2005) *The National Service Framework for Long-term Conditions*. DoH, London.

Dr Foster (2003) *Adult Chronic Pain Management Services in the UK*. Research project in consultation with the Pain Society. Available at www.britishpainsociety.org/pub_pub.html, accessed October 2005.

Fagerhaugh, S.Y. & Strauss, A.L. (1977) *Politics of Pain Management: Staff–Patient Interaction.* Addison-Wesley, San Francisco.

Ferrell, B. (2005) Ethical perspectives on pain and suffering. *Pain Management Nursing* **6**, 3. Available at www.medscape.com/viewarticle/512438, accessed October 2005.

Field, M.J. & Cassel, C.K. (eds) (1997) *Approaching Death: Improving Care at the End of Life.* Committee on Care at the End of Life, Division of Health Care Services, Institute of Medicine. National Academy Press, Washington, DC.

Fine, P.G. (1999) Low-dose ketamine in the management of opioid non-responsive terminal cancer pain. *Journal of Pain and Symptom Management* **17**, 296–300.

Gilson, A.M., Maurer, M.A. & Joranson, D.E. (2005) State policy affecting pain management: recent improvements and the positive impact of regulatory health policies. *Health Policy* **74**, 192–204. Available at www.medsch.wisc.edu/painpolicy/publicat/05hlthpol/05hlthpol.pdf, accessed October 2005.

Higginson, I., Finlay, I., Goodwin, D., et al. (2003) Is there evidence that palliative care teams alter end-of-life experiences of patients and their caregivers? *Journal of Pain and Symptom Management* **25** (2), 150–168.

Manias, E., Botti, M. & Bucknall, T. (2002) Observation of pain assessment and management – the complexities of clinical practice. *Journal of Clinical Nursing* **11**, 724–733.

McCleod, G.A. (2002) The use of audit in acute pain services: a UK perspective. *Acute Pain* **4**, 57–64.

McDonnell, A., Nicholl, J. & Read, S. (2003) Acute pain teams in England: current provision and their role in postoperative pain management. *Journal of Advanced Nursing* **12** (3), 387–393.

Nguyen, M., Ugarte, C., Fuller, I., Haas, G. & Portenoy, R. (2005) Access to care for chronic pain: racial and ethic differences. *The Journal of Pain* **6** (5), 301–314.

Nicholas, M. (2004) When to refer to a pain clinic. *Best Practice and Research Clinical Rheumatology* **18** (4), 613–629.

Nursing and Midwifery Council (2004) *Code of Professional Conduct: Standards for Conduct, Performance and Ethics.* NMC, London. Available at www.nmc-uk.org/aframedisplay.aspx?documentid=201.

Royal College of Surgeons of England and College of Anaesthetists (1990) *Commission on the Provision of Surgical Services.* Report of the Working Party on Pain After Surgery. Royal College of Surgeons of England, London.

Seymour, J., Clark, D. & Winslow, M. (2005) Pain and palliative care: the emergence of new specialties. *Journal of Pain and Symptom Management* **29** (1), 2–13.

Tarzian, A.J. & Hoffman, D.E. (2005) Barriers to managing pain in the nursing home: barriers to a statewide survey. *Journal of the American Medical Directors Association* **6**, S13–S19.

Van Niekerk, L.M. & Martin, F. (2003) The impact of the nurse–physician relationship on barriers encountered by nurses during pain management. *Pain Management Nursing* **4** (1), 3–10.

Watt-Watson, J., Hunter, J. & Pennefather, P. (2004) An integrated undergraduate pain curriculum, based on IASP curricula, for six health science faculties. *Pain* **110**, 140–148.

Wilson, A., Grimshaw, R., Baker, R. & Thompson, J. (1999) Differentiating between audit and research: postal survey of health authorities' views. *British Medical Journal* **319** (7219), 1235.

World Health Organization (1996) *Guidelines: Cancer Pain Relief*, 2nd edn. WHO, Geneva.

World Health Organization (2004) *Palliative Care: Symptom Management and End of Life Care*. WHO, Geneva. Available at http://.whqlibdoc.who.int/hq/2004/who_cds_imai_2004.4.pdf, accessed October 2005.

Index

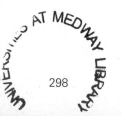